Get Off the Couch
Before It's Too Late

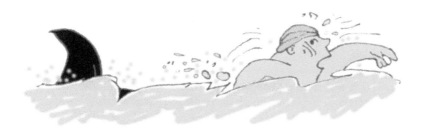

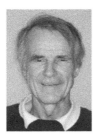

Hugh Bethell MBE MD FRCP FRCGP qualified in medicine in 1966. His early career included a stint as a Cardiac Registrar at Charing Cross Hospital in London, where he first encountered the use of exercise for treating heart disease – a ground-breaking idea at the time.

In 1974 Hugh abandoned cardiology and entered general practice in Alton in Hampshire. There he set up an exercise programme in the Alton Sports Centre for patients recovering from heart attacks and other cardiac ailments and operations. Since then he has written extensively on exercise for heart disease, including two books, nine book chapters, 65 original scientific papers and 76 review articles. In the early 1990s he was the driving force in setting up the British Association for Cardiac Rehabilitation (now the British Association for Cardiac Prevention and Rehabilitation) and became its first President.

Over the past 12 years Hugh has expanded the Cardiac Rehab activities to embrace people with other problems, particularly those that increase the risk of coronary disease – high blood pressure, obesity, diabetes et al. He has also become particularly interested in the exercise treatment of degenerative diseases, disability and frailty in later life, all of which are promoted by an inactive lifestyle. His aim is to encourage regular physical activity for all for disease prevention, increased longevity and, most of all, for a healthy and enjoyable old age.

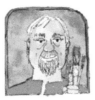

Toni Goffe studied illustration and fine art at Southampton College of Art, where he developed an interest in cartooning at the end of his fourth year. After graduating he moved to London, where he embarked on a career as a freelance cartoonist. Later he began illustrating children's books and worked in this field for many years. On retiring he renewed his enthusiasm for painting and during the lockdown of 2019 returned to his first love, adding cartooning to his weekly routine.

Hugh Bethell used to be Toni's doctor and invited him to illustrate this book. His cartoons appear throughout these pages, in the hope that they will bring a smile or two to the serious subject of exercise.

Get Off the Couch
Before It's Too Late

All the Whys and Wherefores of Exercise

Hugh Bethell

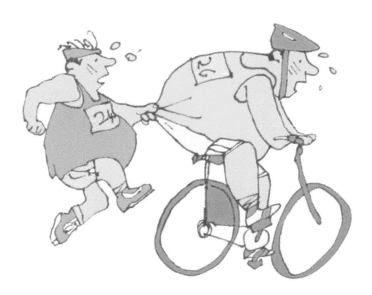

Illustrated by Toni Goffe

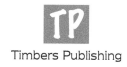

Timbers Publishing

Also by Hugh Bethell
Exercise-based Cardiac Rehabilitation

with Sally Turner
Management and Rehabilitation of the Post-infarct Patient

First published 2021 by Timbers Publishing
Timbers, Boyneswood Road, Medstead GU34 5DY

Text copyright Hugh Bethell 2021
Illustrations copyright Toni Goffe 2021

A catalogue record for this book is available from the British Library

ISBN (paperback) 978-1-7399659-9-0
ISBN (ebook) 978-1-7399659-1-4

Edited by Brenda Updegraff
Design and layout by Robert Updegraff

Printed and bound in Great Britain by IngramSpark

Contents

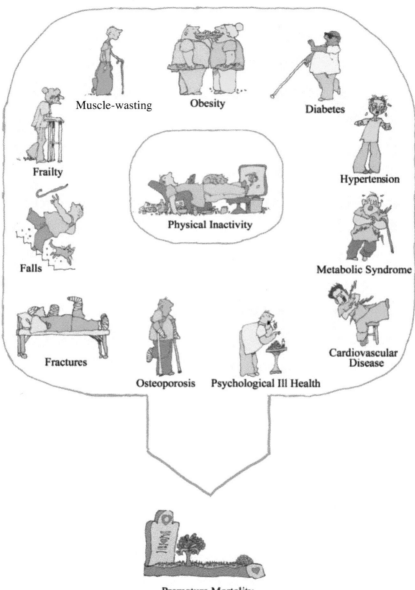

Muscle-wasting

Obesity

Diabetes

Frailty

Hypertension

Physical Inactivity

Falls

Metabolic Syndrome

Fractures

Osteoporosis   Psychological Ill Health

Cardiovascular Disease

Premature Mortality

Preface

I am delighted to write a brief preface for this excellent, informative and entertaining book. You may know me via appearances on television, mainly with my friend Kirstie Allsopp in our long-running series *Location, Location, Location* and *Love It or List It*. What you may not know is that I am an avid exerciser in all its forms. I may work in front of a camera making television for a living – but I am rarely found on the couch in front of it! If I can find a reason to be outdoors running, riding a horse, walking my dogs, bicycling on road or track, skiing, playing cricket or golf, gardening, mountain climbing, canoeing, sailing, then that's where you'll find me . . . and when location or weather don't enable any of these then, yes, I might well be watching television – in the gym at home!

I have also relished taking part in various endurance challenges to raise money and awareness for my favourite charities.

I am certainly no athlete, and could only ever claim to be just about adequate in any of these activities; however, with all this 'movement' going on in my life, I absolutely have experienced the personal benefits of regular exercise – well-being, good physical and mental health, ease with most activities, maintaining a normal body weight, as well as so far managing to swerve any of those nasty diseases which come from being too sedentary. There's simply no better feeling than feeling fit.

Get Off the Couch is a comprehensive guide to all you need to know about physical activity – the mechanics and physiology of exercise; how much we do and how much we should do; how fit we are and how fit we should be; the myriad diseases in later life that can be prevented and treated by exercise; together with the huge benefits of maintaining our physical fitness, particularly into old age. Indeed, according to Hugh Bethell, it is during our later years that the power of exercise becomes most obvious and most essential.

The Covid pandemic has brought home to us all the importance of keeping fit in middle and old age. The grim reaper has scythed through enormous numbers of older people. The most important risk factors for these victims have been obesity and poor mobility – both readily preventable by an appropriately healthy lifestyle, exemplified by keeping physically fit.

So may this book be a wake-up call for those who lead lives with too much sedentary time and too little physical-activity time. Get off the couch – before it is too late. You know it makes sense and I thoroughly support it.

Phil Spencer

Introduction

This book is about physical activity/exercise/sport – what it is, what it does to you, how it is measured and, most of all, what benefits it brings you. It is not a book about particular types of exercise. You will not learn about different exercise regimes, what sport you should take up, whether you should do crunches or press-ups, how to develop a six-pack. There are plenty of books that answer these questions. What I am offering here is information about the science of exercise and how much it has to contribute to our well-being.

The main message of the book is that exercise is essential for a long and healthy life, and for the avoidance of all the degenerative diseases that assail us towards the end of our days. Heart disease, diabetes, osteoporosis, dementia and many other debilitating disorders can be prevented or reduced by regular exercise. These are the conditions that can make later life a misery and lead to the frailty and dependency that are such a burden in our autumn years.

The average time spent with some form of preventable disease at the end of life is about 20 per cent of total lifespan. With an active lifestyle this should be no more than 5 per cent. Being physically fit extends lifespan, but more importantly and to an even greater extent it extends 'healthspan'. It reduces the period of debility at the end of life. It is no coincidence that the level of physical fitness in older people was a factor in whether or not they survived infection with Covid-19. An alternative title for the book might be 'How Not to Kill Granny'.

I hope that this book will become essential reading for all those who would benefit from being more physically active – i.e. nearly everyone! It is particularly aimed at those of you who take too little exercise and need both to recognise that fact and to understand the importance of becoming more active. For you, the dangers of inactivity and the huge benefits of physical activity are set out clearly.

As a medical practitioner, I have been using exercise as medicine for half a century – but the more I learn about the benefits of regular exercise and physical fitness for health, the more I think I should have used it to an even greater extent. The evidence for the importance of exercise rather than pills in the prevention of disease and the maintenance of a long and healthy life is growing by the day. There is now even a medical group to represent this view – the British Association of Lifestyle Medicine. The recognition of the fact that lifestyle trumps medication is dawning on the medical profession and public alike – albeit rather slowly! I hope that this book will help to speed that process.

Hugh Bethell, October 2021

– 1 –

A Very Brief History of Exercise

Holding an Olympic Games means evoking history.
Pierre de Coubertin, founder of the International Olympic Committee

Animals need to move to survive and higher life forms, so-called vertebrates, have evolved muscles and bones for this purpose. These, together with tendons and ligaments, make up the musculoskeletal system. Each animal has developed to suit its own survival needs – the cheetah has a system designed for speed to enable it to catch its prey and likewise the antelope has a system designed for speed to escape being eaten by the cheetah. For other species strength may be more important than speed. Think of the tiger, which can tear its prey limb from limb. For every animal there is a best possible, or 'optimal', mixture of speed and strength to enable it to survive and procreate efficiently.

Evolution has given humans a musculoskeletal system of great versatility. We are neither immensely strong nor immensely fast – but we do have the greatest intelligence in the animal kingdom and we use our brain power to make the most efficient use of this versatility. Man evolved to be a highly efficient hunter-gatherer – to hunt animals and to gather edible plants for our sustenance. For most of human history that has been the main function of our muscles. Primitive man took a lot of exercise because that is what he had to do to survive.

We do not know what prehistoric man did in the way of recreational exercise, though it is likely that during periods of relaxation he would have played around and perhaps danced. There is evidence that in the Palaeolithic age (roughly 2.5 million–10,000 years BC) exercise played a part in social activities and inter-tribe visits.[1] Hunting wild animals allowed the need for food and clothing to blend with recreational sport. We see traces of this today in the activities of some Amazonian tribes who incorporate conversation and singing into their hunting rituals. In today's so-called developed world, the emphasis has been reversed. Fishing and shooting provide recreation first and food very much second, while in fox hunting the need to eat the famously inedible spoils of the hunt has been dispensed with altogether.

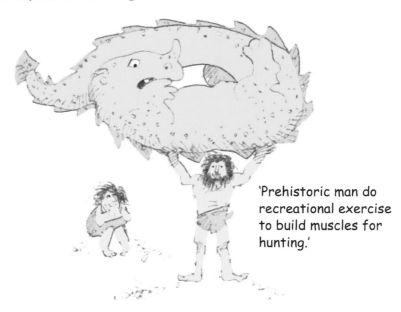

'Prehistoric man do recreational exercise to build muscles for hunting.'

About 10,000 years ago the development of a structured society, a more settled population and the growth of agriculture changed the pattern of human exercising to the more repetitive work associated with husbanding animals and sowing, growing and harvesting crops. With a more secure food source, there would have been more spare time for fun, with games and sports helping muscles to stay in shape even when not so vital for survival. Early forms of organised exercise would also have been used to keep the tribe in battle-ready physical shape; games recorded by the ancient Egyptians and Greeks laid emphasis on activities that would have contributed to this. Egyptian pharaonic carvings and paintings show sports including javelin-throwing, running, swimming, wrestling, rowing and even a primitive form of hockey. Running is specifically recorded as one way of increasing readiness for battle and included distances of up to 96km (60 miles). The original Olympic Games were staged in 776 BC and included running, jumping, discus-throwing, wrestling, boxing, chariot-racing and the first pentathlon. For the Greeks and Romans exercise was also regarded as part of the culture of attaining physical perfection and as an aid to good education – *Mens sana in corpore sano* (A healthy mind in a healthy body).[2]

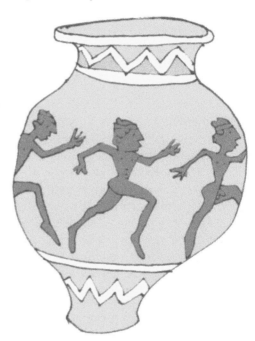

Although exercise at this time would have been a means to an end for contestants, I suspect that such sports would have mainly been pastimes of the strong, the fast and the talented. Even so, several early civilisations recognised exercise as an admirable pursuit, including China with t'ai chi and India with yoga. Running was a prominent feature of religious and daily life for the Kenyan Masai and the Native Americans. Several Greek physicians, including

Greek vase, c.500 BC

Hippocrates (c.460–370 BC) and Galen (c.AD 129–210), extolled the preventative therapeutic benefits of physical activity: 'Eating alone will not keep a man well; he must also take exercise.' However, the idea of the general public taking exercise to maintain health and fitness is a relatively recent phenomenon. I doubt whether the average ancient Greek or Roman citizen would have performed recreational exercise as an aid to improving physical fitness.

The collapse of the Roman Empire in the fourth century AD and the arrival of the 'Dark Ages' saw an end to the culture of the body beautiful. The spread of Christianity brought a belief that the body is sinful – it was the mind and preparation for the afterlife that predominated – though physical fitness remained very much a necessity for the peasants who laboured in the fields and at their various crafts. Hunting was popular with the upper classes and was regarded as a form of work, bringing food to the table. If they exercised otherwise, it was to be prepared for the exertions of combat. As the Middle Ages advanced, jousting became another pastime for the rich. The common man, meanwhile, took to wrestling and early forms of ball games.

An illustration of the extent to which popular recreation expanded in the Middle Ages is to be found in Pieter Brueghel the Elder's painting of children at play, *Children's Games* (1560). More than 90 different children's games are depicted, including sledging, skating, leapfrog, archery and tug of war. Many medieval activities have survived. Among games with a modern equivalent was tennis, perhaps first played with the hand in the 12th century but which has been a racket sport since the 16th century. So-called 'real' or 'royal' tennis was commonplace across the courts of Europe in the 1500s, but we know from Shakespeare's *Henry V* that it was played at least a hundred years before then. Football has been played since the 15th century and cricket since the 16th century.

The Renaissance brought not only a rebirth of academic and other cerebral pursuits but, to a lesser extent, a recognition that the body was more than a mortal shell for the mind and soul. In 1553 a Spaniard, Cristóbal Méndez, published a book on gymnastics entitled *Libro del exercicio corporal y de sus prouechos* (*Book of Physical Exercise and Its Benefits*), while in 1569 an Italian, Girolamo Mercuriale, extended the uses of exercise into the management of disease by natural methods in his book *De Arte Gymnastica*.

The next stage in the advance of recreational exercise came in the late 18th and early 19th centuries with the Industrial Revolution. Up to this time most of the population was still dependent on physical activity to earn the daily crust. The mechanisation of many manual tasks meant that for the first time in history a large proportion of the population no longer had to exercise as part of their gainful employment.

Over the ensuing two centuries the lessening of necessary physical activity has progressed and, since the advent of the motor car and later the computer, has accelerated. Between 1995 and 2014 the proportion of less active occupations rose from 55 per cent to 67 per cent, while the proportion of more active occupations fell from 43 per cent to 33 per cent. 'Less active occupations' include managers, professionals, clerks, technicians, sales and service workers. 'More active occupations' include agriculture, construction, manufacturing, industry and labouring.[3] A survey of the nation's fitness carried out by Allied Dunbar in 1992 estimated that about 80 per cent of men and 90 per cent of women were in occupations that were neither vigorous nor even moderately active.[4]

Today some 75 per cent of jobs are sedentary or require only light physical activity. The graph below shows the inexorable reduction of exercise-based occupations in Westernised societies over the past five decades.[5]

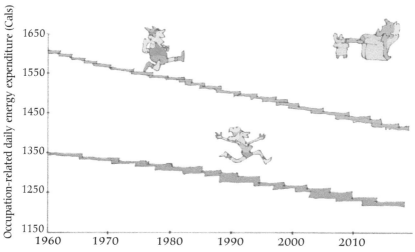

Change in occupational energy expenditure in Westernised societies since 1960

Since the Industrial Revolution there has been an increase in the number of organisations encouraging exercise for the sake of fitness. Initially, in both Europe and the USA, this was based on gymnastics. Competitive games and other sports followed and became increasingly popular – and in 1896 the Olympic Games were revived. Sports included were athletics, cycling, fencing, swimming, gymnastics, sailing, shooting, tennis, weightlifting and wrestling. More recently there has been a progressive increase in the provision of community exercise facilities, with gyms now being a standard facility of hotels and many clubs. At the same time, the cult of competitive sports has also grown and the top players and clubs have attracted enormous devoted fan bases and equally enormous financial rewards.

Paradoxically, the populations of developed nations have become less and less fit, and fatter and fatter. We have divided ourselves into those who exercise and those who spectate. The movement for exercise has certainly attracted many people, but has failed to entrap the majority. Several population surveys have confirmed this sad fact. As one commentator put it: 'Today's interest in sport is more often vicarious than participatory. We idolize the elite athlete who performs for us, rather than the everyday athlete we could and should become.'[6]

Another factor in reducing physical activity in the population has been childhood behaviour. The exercise habit should start early in life. The young of all mammals have a tendency to play – they just frolic and muck about for general enjoyment and the display of high spirits. This leads to the development of the exercise habit, which, because it is fun, influences how grown-ups use their spare time later in life. There has been a dramatic change over the past few decades. First came motorised transport so that children did not need to walk or cycle to get to school and elsewhere. Then came the change in emphasis to more narrow academic demands at school, with less play time and the selling off of playing fields for building. The spread of television meant less outdoor play. The final nail in the coffin of the exercise habit has been the inexorable rise in the time that children spend on their 'screens' – those highly addictive devices that can occupy so much of their leisure time.

A fit and regularly exercising population would have tremendous benefits for the physical, mental, social and financial health of the nation. We will now explore that by looking at the physiology of exercise, the effects of lethargy and exercise, the effects of physical training and the relationship of exercise to disease and longevity.

– 2 –

The Muscles and Types of Exercise

I go for two kinds of men. The kind with muscles
and the kind without. Mae West

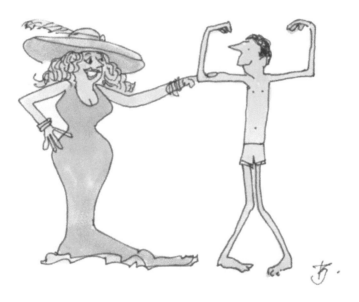

Those of a nervous disposition and those who are easily bored may wish to skip most of this chapter – it describes the internal workings of the muscles, but may not seem particularly important information for the average exerciser. You should, though, be interested in the inheritance pattern of different muscle types and how this determines which exercise will suit you best (see page 21). Beware, however, of skipping Chapter 3 about oxygen transport and the fuelling of exercise – that is vital information.

The muscles are the body's engines – all movement depends on muscular contraction and relaxation. All joints and limbs are powered by muscular contraction and the physiology of muscle action – in other words, the way in which they work – is both beautiful and elegant.

Muscle types

Your muscles are divided into three distinct varieties:

1. Voluntary muscles. These are also called skeletal or 'striated' muscles (because of their stripy appearance under the microscope). Their movements are under our control – like, say, the biceps. Think that you want to bend your arm, put it into action and, hey presto, you contract your biceps and your arm bends.

2. Involuntary muscles. These are also called 'smooth' muscles. They perform the vital activities of the body over which we have no control. They just get on with it, like the muscles of the gut which labour away moving food down the gastrointestinal tract. Or the ocular muscles which control the pupil: they respond to light but not to any conscious thought process.

3. Cardiac muscle. The heart is a very specialised form of involuntary muscle which we will meet in some detail later.

Our main concern in this book will be with the voluntary muscles, the muscles of movement. They have a main body, the belly of the muscle, and very strong fibrous cables called tendons that attach the muscle to the bones. Most movements depend on muscles contracting, bending or straightening the joints that connect the bones to which the tendons are attached.

Each muscle is made up of thousands of fibres, which in turn are made up of thousands of myofibrils, tubular structures extending the whole length of the cell. The myofibrils are made up of thick and thin filaments; the thick filaments are composed mainly of myosin and the thin filaments of actin.

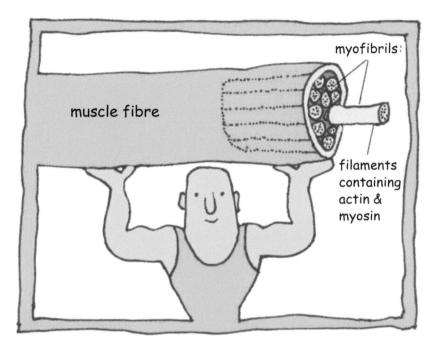

myofibrils

muscle fibre

filaments containing actin & myosin

Muscle contraction is stimulated by an impulse passing down the nerve supplying the muscle – the motor neuron (I won't bore you with the physiology of this process; suffice it to say that its effect is similar to the arrival of an electrical impulse). Each muscle is served by a large number of nerve fibres and the individual motor neuron plus the muscle fibres that it stimulates is called a motor unit. When an impulse reaches the muscle fibres of a motor unit, it stimulates a reaction between the actin and myosin filaments. This reaction results in the start of a contraction, which is achieved by the two different types of filament sliding alongside each other causing the whole muscle to shorten. Viewed under a microscope the muscle fibres have a striped appearance – hence striated muscle – which is caused by the highly ordered arrangement of the actin and myosin within the fibrils and the similarly ordered arrangement of the fibrils within the muscle cell.

Contraction continues until the neuron stops stimulating the muscle, or until muscle fatigue sets in. This happens when the supply of energy that fuels contraction is exhausted.

One more important fact about muscles. They are made up of two distinct types of fibre – slow-twitch (Type I) and fast-twitch (Type II) fibres (which are further subdivided into Type IIa and Type IIb fibres). Slow-twitch fibres contract slowly and can maintain their shortening for long periods – they are the strength- and endurance-giving fibres and are particularly used during such activities as distance running and cycling. Fast-twitch fibres contract rapidly but tire quickly and are those most used by sprinters and weightlifters. Repeated contractions give speed to action.

Most muscles consist of a combination of slow- and fast-twitch fibres, but one often predominates in particular muscles – for instance, back muscles, which move little but contract continuously to maintain posture, are predominantly slow-twitch. Eye muscles, on the other hand, are almost all fast-twitch. There is also a genetic influence on the predominance and distribution of muscle type. The ratio of slow to fast is about 50 per cent for most of us. However, some individuals inherit a much larger proportion of one or the other and that may determine their prowess in different sporting endeavours. Those born with a higher proportion of Type I slow-twitch fibres are more likely to become endurance athletes, while those born with more Type II fast-twitch fibres will do better as sprinters. Specialist training can change the balance somewhat but a born marathon runner will never make a champion sprinter.

Exercising your muscles

This is not a book about which particular type of exercise you could or should be taking – my message is just do it, whatever you like. Exercise is more likely to be sustained if you enjoy it, so choose carefully.

There are two broad categories of exercise. **Dynamic or isotonic exercise** is that which uses the regular, purposeful movement of joints and large muscle groups, particularly their Type I fibres. **Isometric exercise**, on the other hand, involves static contraction of muscles with little or no joint movement, predominantly involving Type II fibres. Other ways of describing types of exercise include aerobic (using oxygen) and anaerobic (not needing oxygen). Most activities involve a combination of these factors and classification is typically determined by the dominant characteristics of the particular exercise.

Aerobic/dynamic exercise

Dynamic or aerobic exercise includes such sports as running, cycling, swimming and aerobic dance. These involve much movement and little strength and can be continued for long periods; they are sometimes also referred to as 'cardiovascular' workouts. They are dependent on a good supply of oxygen, which fuels the energy produced by the breakdown of carbohydrate into glucose and stored in the muscle as glycogen. Such exercise,

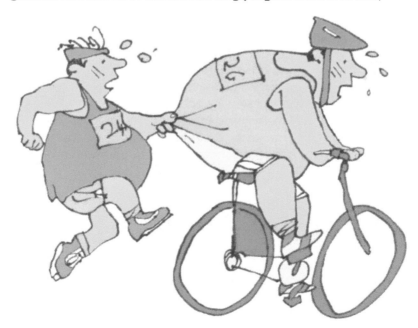

performed at the right level, can be continued as long as there is a sufficient supply of glycogen. If the duration and intensity of the exercise is sufficient to deplete the glycogen faster than it can be replenished, muscle fatigue sets in and the exercise must be greatly reduced or stopped. This is the experience of the marathon runner who 'hits the wall'. The effort of aerobic exercise is mainly performed by Type I, or slow-twitch, muscle fibres.

Most of the clinical benefits of exercise in preventing and treating chronic diseases have been demonstrated for aerobic exercise and it is this form of exercise that is the main subject of this book.

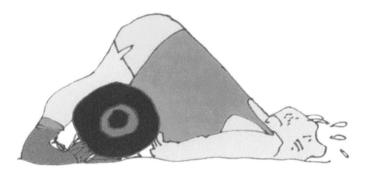

Isometric exercise

Anaerobic or isometric exercise involves much strength but little movement. More mature readers will remember the once well-known Charles Atlas muscle-building techniques. These were pure isometrics, involving one muscle group straining against another without movement – a form of exertion designed to build up muscle bulk. The muscle fibres used are the Type II, or fast-twitch, fibres. They do not use oxygen and they tire quickly. Most so-called anaerobic exercises do involve some movement but make much more use of strength. Examples are weightlifting and sprinting. In a clinical context, isometric exercise is frequently used by physiotherapists in the treatment of joint injuries and after orthopaedic surgery. Muscle-strengthening is also very important in the treatment of frailty and balance problems in old age – both of which will be discussed later.

Nearly all exercise involves a mixture of aerobic and isometric effort, though one or the other usually predominates. Most gym fitness-training programmes use a mixture and the recommendations of the Department of Health include doing 'strengthening activities that work all the major muscles [legs, hips, back, abdomen, chest, shoulders and arms] on at least 2 days a week' – see Chapter 6.

In the gym you will find a number of exercise types on offer. These are some examples:

- **Cardiovascular** – this includes mainly aerobic exercise such as using a static bike or rowing machine, walking or running on a treadmill, skipping, aerobic dance and any other exercise designed to raise the heart rate and make you thoroughly short of breath.

- **Bums and tums** – aimed mainly at young to middle-aged women concerned about their body image, this consists of a mixture of aerobic and isometric exercise concentrating on the abdomen, buttocks and thighs. Crunches, squats and jogging may be included.

- **Pilates** – an exercise system involving a mixture of mental concentration, economy of movement, building up core strength and breathing control. This may use free-standing exercise or weights and pulleys.

- **BODYBALANCE**™ – uses a mixture of yoga, t'ai chi and Pilates to improve core strength, relax the mind and enhance flexibility.

- **Spinning** – group cycling under the direction of an instructor who changes the load and speed through the session; mainly aerobic.

- **Aquarobics** – exercise in the swimming pool that uses the resistance of the water to exercise different muscle groups and may be particularly suitable for those with lower-limb problems, who can be helped by the support provided by the flotation environment and who would be unable to exercise without support.

- **Calisthenics** – a variety of body movements, often rhythmical, generally without using equipment or apparatus, thus in essence bodyweight training. The exercises are intended to increase body strength, body fitness and flexibility through movements such as pulling or pushing oneself up, bending, jumping or swinging, using only one's body weight for resistance.

- **Zumba** – a form of aerobic dance with varying rhythms and intensity which can be adapted to all age groups.

- **Boxercise** – an exercise based on the training concepts that boxers use to keep fit. Classes can take a variety of formats but a typical one may involve shadow-boxing, skipping, hitting pads, kicking punchbags, press-ups, shuttle-runs and sit-ups.

The possible combinations of exercise are infinite and the effects of one form compared with another depend on the balance of aerobic, isometric and flexibility exercises. They are all good, so if you want to use the gym and don't find it too boring, just choose that or those which you will enjoy. There is no greater disincentive to sticking with a programme than not wanting to be there! And there is no evidence that one sort of exercise class is any better or worse than any other – whatever individual adherents may say.

If you wish to make up your own circuit, I suggest that you alternate the stations between 'cardiovascular' and 'MSE – muscular strength and endurance'. You don't need to go to a gym to do this – you can do it at home with the help of your staircase or an aerobic step, a pair of dumbbells or 'TheraBands' – thick elastic bands for straining against. Overleaf you will find a sample of what might be possible.

My personal preference is for competitive sports or outdoor exercise. Team sports have the disadvantage of having to find a number of like-minded individuals to join you; you probably need to belong to a specific sports club. Running, swimming and cycling can be performed in groups or on your own and

Home Exercises

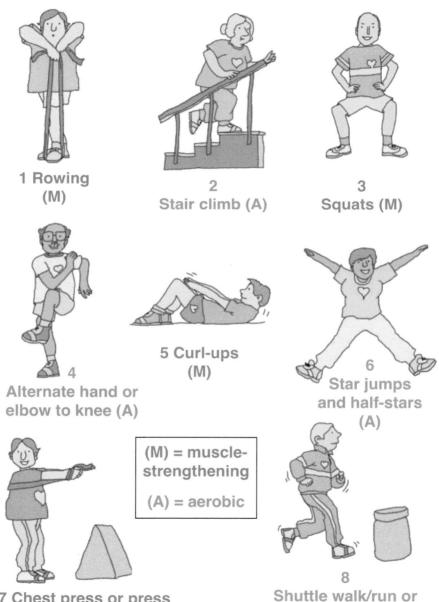

1 Rowing (M)

2 Stair climb (A)

3 Squats (M)

4 Alternate hand or elbow to knee (A)

5 Curl-ups (M)

6 Star jumps and half-stars (A)

(M) = muscle-strengthening

(A) = aerobic

7 Chest press or press against a wall (M)

8 Shuttle walk/run or walk/run on the spot (A)

have the great convenience that they can be fitted in with whatever else is going on in your life. Just choose what exercise(s) suit you best and which you enjoy enough to want to continue in the long term. If it gets you moving and out of breath, it is doing the business.

Warming up and cooling down

For any exercise you are almost always advised to warm up before starting – for anything from a few minutes to half an hour. This is received wisdom for exercise professionals and if you take part in a supervised exercise class the warm-up is an integral part of the session. The purpose is to loosen up and warm the joints, muscles and tendons, making them more flexible and ready for exercise, and thus less vulnerable to injury. It certainly sounds like something sensible to do, but in fact there is little evidence to support it. If you have a choice, avoid spending too much time on warming up – if you have limited time for exercising, don't waste time on the preliminaries. And you can always start slowly and use this as your warm-up.

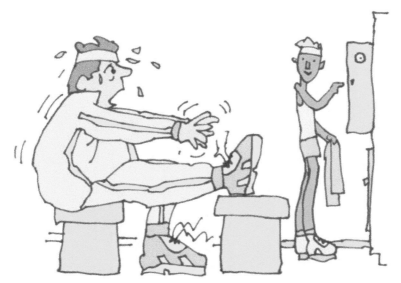

'I'm not doing warming-up exercises. I'm trying to reach my laces!'

Cooling down, however, is more valuable and really can prevent problems. At the end of a session you are likely to be hot and sweaty with your blood vessels dilated. If you just stand about at this stage your heart rate falls but your blood vessels tend to remain dilated to promote heat loss. As a result, your blood pressure falls, which may cause you to feel faint or even keel over – not dangerous, but preventable by cooling down. It is advisable to keep moving until your blood vessels have contracted enough to prevent the fall in blood pressure.

Another commonly promoted preliminary to taking exercise is stretching. Again the idea is to prepare the muscles and tendons for the more violent changes about to be brought on by exercise. There are two forms of stretch – static and dynamic. Both are beloved by exercise professionals, but they too have very little evidence to support them.[1] Indeed it has been shown that static calf muscle stretches actually *increase* the risk of injury among runners, perhaps by reducing the strength in the stretched muscles.[2] Although there is some evidence that performance may be slightly improved by dynamic warm-up, for my money it is tiring and not worth the candle – I would rather just get on with it.

Oxygen as the Fuel of Exercise

People say you can't live without love, but I think oxygen is more important.
Anon.

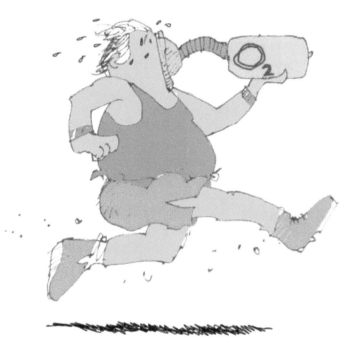

That's enough about muscles for the time being – but we will hear a bit more about them later. This chapter is about the role of oxygen in fuelling exercise. It is a very important topic and knowing about it helps you to understand the benefits of exercise as well as how it is measured and prescribed.

For a muscle to work it needs energy and energy requires fuel. The biochemical processes that fuel muscle contraction are immensely complicated – much too complicated to go into in detail here – except for the contribution of oxygen (O_2). Oxygen is an essential component of the metabolic conversion of various energy sources (sugars, fats, etc.) into action – in other words, muscle contraction. The supply of oxygen to the muscle and the muscle's use of it are the factors that decide how much work that muscle can perform during aerobic exercise.

Oxygen makes up about 20 per cent of the air we breathe and it is absorbed from the lungs on to the haemoglobin molecules in the blood's red cells as they pass through the very small blood vessels (capillaries) supplying the air sacs (alveoli) in the lungs. Haemoglobin arrives in the lungs in the form of deoxyhaemoglobin and has a bluish hue. The oxygen picked up in the lungs converts it to oxyhaemoglobin, which is a much brighter red. The blood is pumped round the body to the various organs that need oxygen to maintain life – the brain, heart, kidneys, gut, liver and muscles of the respiration system. There the oxygen is extracted into the cells. On average, oxygen uptake at rest is about 3.5ml of oxygen per minute per kilogram of body weight, meaning that for a 70kg (11 stone) resting man the rate of oxygen consumption would be about 250ml per minute. This is also known as 1 MET. Remember the term MET – it stands for metabolic equivalent and it is an extremely important measure of exercise intensity.

When we exercise, our muscles need more oxygen and this is provided by breathing faster and by the heart pumping more blood to them. There is a straight-line relationship between muscle work and oxygen uptake (abbreviated as VO_2) until the point at which no more oxygen can be absorbed and pumped round the body – known as the maximum oxygen uptake, or VO_{2max}. This is measured as millilitres of oxygen used per minute for each kilogram of body weight – ml/min/kg. This is aerobic exercise and at the point of maximum uptake further exercise can only continue using anaerobic (not using oxygen) metabolism. This is fuelled by stored energy sources in the muscles which quickly become used up. Anaerobic exercise can therefore be continued for only a very short period.

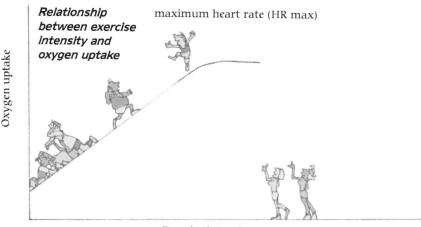

Relationship between exercise intensity and oxygen uptake

maximum heart rate (HR max)

Oxygen uptake

Exercise intensity

As exercise workload increases, so does oxygen uptake to the point of exhaustion. For the unfit, this point is reached at a lower oxygen uptake and therefore a lower workload than for the fit individual. The fitter you are, the higher the rate at which you can take up and use oxygen and therefore the higher the workload you can achieve – as illustrated in the following graph of exertion against oxygen uptake.

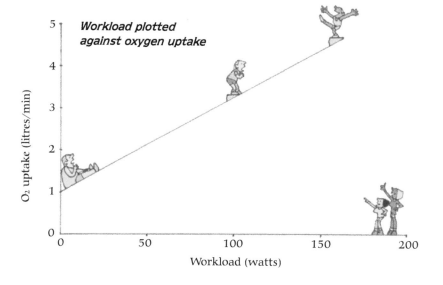

Workload plotted against oxygen uptake

O_2 uptake (litres/min)

Workload (watts)

The concept of VO_{2max} is very important. It is the most precise measure of physical fitness we have, since it describes the maximum work rate of which a person is capable. In healthy young people it is usually between 35 and 55ml/min/kg body weight (10–15 METs). Ultra-fit athletes may reach levels of 70–80ml/min/kg, or 20–23 METs. Heart patients tend to have much lower levels, in the range of 10–30ml/min/kg. As we age there is a decline in VO_{2max} of roughly 0.5–1.0ml/min/kg each year after our late teens or early twenties. However, the variation in individual VO_{2max} is far greater than the age variation.

Exercise to VO_{2max} can be attained only by using the large muscle groups of the legs. Because of their smaller bulk, maximum arm exercise will achieve only about two thirds of maximum leg exercise. Also, once maximum oxygen uptake has been reached with leg exercise, bringing other muscles, like the arm muscles, into action will not increase oxygen uptake further. The limiting factor is not muscular effort but the ability of the lungs and heart to supply oxygen to the muscles.

Oxygen transport during exercise

From the resting state to exercise, the increase in oxygen uptake and transport is achieved by several changes:

- **Ventilation, or breathing** Faster and deeper breathing brings more oxygen into contact with the capillary blood in the air sacs in the lungs. For people without lung disease, the saturation of oxygen in the blood does not fall with exercise, indicating that breathing and the lungs are not the limiting factor for exercise or for VO_{2max}.

- **Cardiac output, or the amount of blood pumped out by the heart** At rest the normal heart rate (HR) is about 70 beats per minute. With each heartbeat about 70–80ml of blood is pumped into the circulation – this is the stroke volume (SV). So the volume pumped out each minute is about 70 x 75, which comes to roughly 5.5 litres per minute – this is the resting cardiac output (CO).

With increasing exercise the CO rises steadily with oxygen uptake to the point of VO_{2max} at which it levels off – at about 20–25 litres per minute. This four- to fivefold increase in cardiac output is mediated by a more than doubling of the heart rate to 180–200 per minute and a less than doubling of stroke volume to about 130ml – i.e. the heart beats more rapidly and pumps out more blood with each stroke. There is a straight-line relationship between increasing heart rate and increasing oxygen uptake.

The fit individual can perform a heavier workload than the unfit at any given heart rate. Since getting fit by exercise training does not change the maximum heart rate, the greater exercise level that can be achieved by the fit individual is mediated by an increase in stroke volume combined with more efficient oxygen use by the muscles (see Chapter 5).

In adults, maximum heart rate is approximately 220 minus age, and reduces gradually with age. So a 20-year-old exercising maximally should reach a HR of about 200, while for a 70-year-old the rate would be around 150.

• **Extraction of blood by the muscles** The arteries supplying the muscles carry a full load of oxygen – the haemoglobin molecules are fully saturated with oxygen. The amount of oxygen extracted from the blood by the muscles depends on how hard the muscles are working. At rest the muscles extract about 5.5ml oxygen for every 100ml of blood flow, rising to about 17ml oxygen during maximal exercise. This is achieved partly by an increased rate of oxygen uptake by each muscle fibre and partly by an increased blood flow to the muscles. Working muscles may use up to 18 times as much oxygen as they do at rest.

One type of muscle involved in exercise, the heart muscle or myocardium, differs from striated, voluntary muscle. Unlike the voluntary muscles, heart muscle extracts as much oxygen from its blood supply as it can at all times – both when 'resting' and when working at full capacity. Therefore the only way in which heart muscle can get more oxygen is by an increase in blood flow. This becomes important for people with narrowing of their coronary arteries (see Coronary Heart Disease, Chapter 10).

- **Combined effect on oxygen uptake** For a young person of average fitness, the increase of VO_2 from rest to maximum exercise is about twelvefold – mediated by a fourfold rise in cardiac output (HR up by 2.7 times and SV up by 1.4 times) and a threefold rise in arteriovenous oxygen difference.

VO_{2max} varies with age, sex and habitual physical activity. As time goes by, maximal heart rate and stroke volume both decline, as do muscle bulk and strength, so that the fall in VO_{2max} each year is between 0.5 and 1 ml/min/kg body weight. Although the older you are the less fit you become, the variation between individuals is much greater than the variation with age – mainly because of the effect of habitual activity. Women, who have smaller frames and smaller hearts than men but more fat, have a VO_{2max} that is about 20 per cent lower than in men. The influence of habitual activity on fitness will be discussed in Chapter 6.

Exercise Dose:
How Much are You Doing?

If you think that a minute goes by really fast
you have never been on a treadmill. Anon.

You might wonder why it can be helpful to regard exercise as a 'dose', let alone measure it. Two reasons pop into my mind:

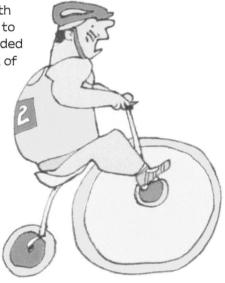

1. Because of its widespread health benefits, exercise can be equated to medication. How big a dose is needed to help control weight, reduce risk of diabetes or lengthen life? What is the dose response – i.e. the ratio between the dose of exercise and the extent of any benefits? What would be the dose required to produce the same life-prolonging effect as, for example, taking a cholesterol-lowering drug like simvastatin at 40mg a day? The answer is never straightforward. For instance, the intensity with which the exercise is performed changes its effect on health. An hour's brisk walking may equate to the same exercise dose as walking about slowly all day, but the effects will be very different.

2. Exercise is on one side of the equation that decides weight change. Comparing the calorie content of our food with the calorie output of our exercise allows us to see why we are getting fatter – and what might help reverse this. For this purpose, the intensity of the exercise should not be important, only the total dose.

There are several ways of expressing the amount of exercise taken and all are related to the oxygen cost of the activity:

• **Rate of exertion** This is the measure of exercise intensity which tells us the rate of oxygen consumption. It can be expressed as an absolute rate – i.e. litres of oxygen per minute (L/min) – or, as we saw in Chapter 3, relative to the exerciser's weight as millilitres of oxygen per minute per kilogram of body weight (ml/min/kg). The weight-related figure is usually divided by 3.5 to give the rate of exertion in METs (metabolic equivalents). An example would be the rate of oxygen consumption required by a 70kg man walking on a treadmill at, say, 4mph – this takes approximately 17ml/min/kg or 4.9 METs and equates to about 1.2 litres of oxygen per minute. The heavier you are, the more effort you need to move yourself along, so for a 100kg man the equivalent figures would still be 17ml/min/kg or 4.9 METs, but this would equate to about 1.7 litres of oxygen per minute. No wonder fat people get more out of breath with exercise than thin people.

• **Total energy expended** This tells us the total oxygen consumed by a particular period of exercise and is the actual dose of exercise taken. In the example given above, if the 70kg man walks at 4mph for 10 minutes he will have consumed 12 litres of oxygen, while the heavier man will have consumed 17 litres. These figures can be converted into calories, or the SI equivalent, joules.

Unfortunately, common usage has made the calorie a more complicated unit than it need be – sorry about this, but you do need to understand what a calorie means. A calorie is the amount of energy (in the form of heat) needed to increase the temperature of 1ml of water by 1 degree centigrade. Since this is such a small amount of energy, nearly everybody works in kilocalories (kcals or Calories – note the capital C), calories multiplied by 1,000. Confusingly, many people call the kcal a calorie! So if you read figures measured in calories, particularly in relation to food, the writer means kcals. It would be a lot simpler if we converted to the metric equivalent, joules, but calories are deeply ingrained in our language and culture, so that is never going to happen. One little calorie is equivalent to about 4.2 joules and one big Calorie or kcal is equivalent to about 4.2 kilojoules (kjoules).

In human physiology, each litre of oxygen used is converted into about 5 Calories of energy or about 21 kjoules. In the cases of our walking men above, in 10 minutes the thinner man has used $12 \times 5 = 60$ Calories or $12 \times 21 = 252$ kjoules. The fatter man has used 85 Calories or 357 kjoules – just work it out. You may find this system useful for assessing the dose of exercise in relation to how much food it takes to fuel a certain amount of effort. I regret to tell you that it takes a disappointingly small quantity of food to fuel enormous efforts! One Mars bar will provide enough energy for 40 minutes of brisk walking at 4mph for the thin man. An often-quoted index of high-calorie food is its equivalence in teaspoonfuls of sugar. A teaspoonful is just slightly over 5ml, which converts to about 4g of sugar, which is worth about 15 Calories.

- Total exercise dose can also be calculated as MET minutes or MET hours.[1] As explained above, a MET, or metabolic equivalent, is the rate at which energy is used by the body at rest. It is expressed in relation to body weight and is taken as 3.5ml of oxygen per minute per kilogram. A 70kg man walking at 4mph will be exercising at about 5 METs. If he maintains this pace for an hour he will have expended $5 \times 60 = 300$ MET minutes. It is not too difficult to calculate the total number of MET minutes of exercise you expend in a week – though it may demand a degree of obsessiveness to do so. Just add up the MET minutes of all the exercise you have done, but remember that the actual energy cost of each exercise is only an approximation. If you are anything like the rest of humanity, this will be an overestimate!

It is then possible to convert the exercise dose from MET minutes into Calories using the formula overleaf:

$$\text{Total MET minutes} \times 3.5 \times \text{body weight in kilograms} \div 200$$
$$= \text{number of Calories used}$$

For example, the 70kg man walking briskly for an hour will have used:
$$5 \times 60 \times 3.5 \times 70 \div 200 = 367.5 \text{ Calories}$$

For health benefits for most adults, the national guidelines suggest using exercise to burn about 900 Calories per week, roughly 150 minutes of brisk walking; for weight loss and even greater health benefits, an expenditure of 1,800 Calories per week or 5 hours' walking.

Unfortunately it is not easy to measure exercise intensity or dose, however we choose to do it or to express it. Very few exercises are sufficiently independent of the effort we put into them, or of our skill in their performance, to use an amount of energy that is more or less the same for everyone. Those that are predictable include walking, cycling and running – on the flat without a wind. For most other exercise we can only give approximations of energy expenditure. For instance, it is possible to give rough estimates of the energy costs of playing tennis or of various gym activities, but they will be very dependent on the amount of effort put into the activity by the performer.

Using modern accelerometer devices (Fitbits and the like) should allow more accurate estimates of the amount of exercise taken, but would rely on heart-rate responses and would need to be calibrated to the individual to produce anything like accurate measures of energy expenditure.

There are endless tables indicating the intensity of different sorts of exercise – usually expressed either as METs required or oxygen cost. None is particularly accurate because the answer depends so much on how hard the exerciser is trying – how hard he or she goes at it. However, they do give an idea of exercise intensity of different activities. Opposite is an example. I have added an idea of the number of Calories used per hour for a 70kg individual.

Physical activity	MET value	VO$_2$ ml/min/kg	Cals/hour Cals/hour
Light-intensity activities	**< 3**		
Sleeping	0.9	3.1	63
Watching television	1.0	3.5	70
Writing, desk work, typing	1.5	5.2	106
Strolling, 1.7mph (2.7km/h), level ground	2.3	8.1	162
Walking, 2.5mph (4km/h)	2.9	10.1	205
Moderate-intensity activities	**3 to 6**		
Stationary bicycling, 50 watts, very light	3.0	10.5	212
Walking, 3mph (4.8km/h)	3.3	11.5	233
Playing golf	3.5	12.2	247
Calisthenics, home exercise, light or moderate effort	3.5	12.2	247
Walking, 3.4mph (5.5km/h)	3.6	12.6	254
Cycling, <10mph (16km/h)	4.0	14.0	282
Doubles tennis	5.0	17.5	353
Heavy gardening	5.5	19.2	388
Stationary bicycling, 100 watts, light	5.5	19.2	388
Sexual activity	5.8	20.3	409
Vigorous-intensity activities	**> 6**		
Jogging	7.0+	24.5+	494
Singles tennis, squash, racketball	7.0–12.0	24.5–42.0	494–847
Calisthenics (e.g. push-ups, sit-ups, pull-ups, star jumps), vigorous effort	8.0	28.0	565
Running on the spot	8.0	28.0	565
Rope skipping	10.0	35.0	706

This table can give only a very rough estimate of the energy cost of these activities – a rough guide to the cost to the average-sized individual making an average effort. More detailed estimates can be found elsewhere.[2] You can also go online for a calculator which will give you the energy cost of walking, running, cycling, skipping and rowing, taking into account your weight, speed and duration of exercise.[3]

The exercise that most people do most of is walking – and very good exercise it is too. Brisk walking is all you need to satisfy the recommendations of the health gurus, so below is a table giving you the exercise intensities of walking at different speeds. The figures given are for walking on the flat with neither a following nor a head wind. The MET values are the same for everyone irrespective of weight. The Calories-consumed column is for a 70kg (11 stone) individual. Lighter people will expend fewer calories and heavier people will expend more, so one advantage of being overweight is that the heavier you are, the easier it *should* be to lose weight.

Speed mph	Mins per mile	METs	VO₂ ml/min/kg	Cals/hour
2.0	30	2.5	8.9	176
2.5	24	2.9	10.2	205
3.0	20	3.3	11.5	233
3.5	17	3.7	12.9	261
3.75	16	4.4	15.3	310
4.0	15	4.9	17.1	346

The relationship between walking speed and oxygen need is a straight line at lower speeds but above 3mph it becomes harder to increase speed – and each increment in speed becomes more costly in terms of oxygen demand. For most people, brisk walking means travelling at between 3 and 4mph.

Jogging/running is the most straightforward form of exercise – it is a highly efficient way of increasing fitness, it is quick to do, needs minimal equipment and expenditure, and does not require an opponent – and even so it can be a most satisfying social occasion. Below are the exercise intensities of running at different speeds. Again, the figures presume the unlikely scenario of no hills and no wind, and the Calorie expenditure is that of an individual weighing 70kg (11 stone).

Speed mph	Mins per mile	METs	VO$_2$ ml/min/kg	Cals/hour
3.5	17 mins	6.4	22.3	451
4.0	15 mins	7.1	24.9	501
4.5	13 mins			
	20 secs	7.9	27.6	558
5.0	12 mins	8.7	30.3	614
5.5	10 mins			
	54 secs	9.4	33	663
6.0	10 mins	10.2	35.7	720
6.5	9 mins			
	13 secs	11	38.3	776
7.0	8 mins			
	34 secs	11.7	41.0	826
7.5	8 mins	12.5	43.7	882
8.0	7 mins			
	30 secs	13.3	46.4	939
8.5	7 mins			
	40 secs	14	49.1	988
9.0	6 mins			
	40 secs	14.8	51.7	1,045
9.5	6 mins			
	19 secs	15.5	54.4	1,094
10.0	6 mins	16.3	57.1	1,150

You will see that running at low speeds is less efficient than walking. If you wish to go at 4mph, walk don't run!

Cycling is another exercise for which it is possible to calculate energy expenditure. Below are the very approximate figures for the MET value, oxygen cost and calorie expenditure for cycling on the flat without wind for a 70kg (11 stone) individual. Real life conditions mean that the energy costs are usually much higher.

Speed mph	METs	VO$_2$ ml/min/kg	Cals/hour
10	5	17.5	470
12	7	24.5	514
14	9	31.5	661
16	11.5	40.2	845
18	14	49.0	1,200

Physical Fitness: the Best Measure of How Much Exercise You Can Do

It's easier to stay in shape if you never let yourself get out of shape in the first place. Bill Loguidice, fitness guru

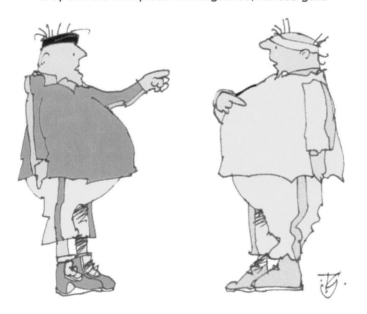

There are several ways to describe your level of physical fitness, including maximum oxygen uptake (VO_{2max}), exercise capacity and aerobic capacity. As we have seen (page 32), VO_{2max} is the standard measure of physical fitness. The level for a young to middle-aged adult averages between 30 and 50ml/min/kg – about 8.5–14 METs.

The increase in VO_{2max} that can be attained by physical training is inversely proportional to the starting VO_{2max}: in other words, the less active you have been, the less fit you are, then the more you have to gain from training. An inactive, unfit person can be improved by a greater percentage than an out-of-training athlete, though not to such a high level. The increase may exceed 30 per cent in young, unfit individuals who begin to train intensively. Older subjects show a smaller response to training than younger ones.

The graph below shows the effects of fitness level on heart rate and oxygen uptake. The fitter you are, the more exercise you can do – i.e. the more oxygen you can absorb and use, for any given heart rate. Since it is the maximum heart rate that limits your ability to exercise maximally, the fitter you are, the greater your maximal effort capacity (see also the illustration on page 31). For most of us for most of the time, however, it is 'submaximal exercise' (exercise at a defined level which is lower than the peak that can be reached) that is more important – few of us exercise maximally, but we all exercise submaximally. In this case, any exercise level for a fit person expends a lower proportion of what is possible – all effort becomes easier.

If you take up a fitness regime you will be able to get an idea of changes in your fitness level by observing the fall in your heart rate (pulse rate) at rest and during exercise.

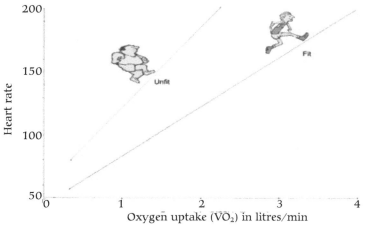

Heart rate v. physical fitness in the fit and unfit individual

The increased aerobic capacity produced by training is brought about by a mixture of 'central' and 'peripheral' effects. Central effects include:

1. Improved cardiac performance After training, the heart is able to contract more efficiently, pumping out a larger volume of blood with each beat. The stroke volume increases. At rest, the body's need for oxygen and therefore cardiac output is the same for the fit as for the unfit person. Since the fit individual pumps out more blood with each beat (the stroke volume) than the unfit, his or her resting heart rate is lower, perhaps as low as 50 beats per minute in the super-fit.

During submaximal exercise, again the need for circulating blood and oxygen delivery is the same in trained and untrained people. So at any given level of exercise the cardiac output is the same for the fit as for the unfit – but the stroke volume is higher and the heart rate is lower for the fit. Submaximal exercise is easier for the fit than for the unfit and achieved with a lower heart rate. Maximal oxygen uptake, however, is increased by physical training. The maximal heart rate does not increase, but cardiac output is greater because stroke volume is greater. More blood and oxygen can be pumped to the working muscles, which can therefore do more work. That is why the fit long-distance runner can run faster than the unfit.

2. Reduced sympathetic tone The resistance to flow in the peripheral blood vessels is partly determined by the 'sympathetic' nervous system – the network of nerves that supply the tiny muscles which can contract and narrow small arteries. Physical training reduces this tone and opens up peripheral arteries, allowing blood to flow more freely through them and reducing blood pressure at rest and during exercise. The heart has to work less hard to pump blood round the system.

3. Changes in blood The trained individual has a greater total blood volume and more oxygen-bearing red cells. 'Blood doping'* relies on this effect to improve the prowess of athletes.

*Blood doping is a technique used by athletes to cheat the system. Blood is taken and stored long before a competition and is then transfused back just prior to the event. This gives the athlete the enhanced advantage of greater blood volume and red cell mass than could be achieved by simple training alone. A similar effect can also be achieved by training at high altitude or by sleeping in a tent with lower oxygen concentration than is found in the atmosphere.

Peripheral effects of physical training include:

1. Increased muscle performance Trained muscles exhibit a number of changes. They become larger, they develop more mitochondria (the enzyme packages within muscle cells that are much concerned with energy production) and they have a better ability to extract oxygen and glucose from the blood.

2. Increased muscle blood flow The larger muscles have a greater network of capillaries feeding them and the distribution of blood flow favours working muscles over inactive muscles.

3. Increased arteriovenous oxygen difference Better muscle performance and more efficient blood flow results in an increase in the overall extraction of oxygen from the blood – the venous blood being carried back to the heart has less oxygen left in it. This is most marked at maximal effort.

Combined central and peripheral effects:

1. In young people the training-induced increase in maximal aerobic capacity is brought about equally by central and peripheral effects. The exact magnitude of the central training effect is related to the size of the muscles being used. Training of leg muscles has a greater effect than training of arm muscles.

Training of one set of muscles will result in increased exercise capacity when a different set of muscles is used, but the improvement is only about half that achieved by exercise with the trained muscles. Elegant experiments have shown that individuals trained in one-legged cycling on an ergometer do show an improved performance with the untrained leg, but this is still much less than that for the trained leg.[1]

2. Older people react rather differently – the central effects of training are less pronounced and the peripheral effects are more important.

Measuring physical fitness

I will start with how the professionals do it – but read on and you will find out how to do it for yourself. For those of you who skipped Chapter 3, let me repeat that the best measure of physical fitness or aerobic capacity is the maximal oxygen uptake or VO_{2max}. However, most methods of measuring physical fitness or aerobic capacity estimate VO_{2max} rather than measuring it directly.

VO_{2max} can be measured directly, but it is a time-consuming business and needs specialised and expensive equipment. It is usually performed on a calibrated bicycle ergometer or on a treadmill. The candidate performs the exercise while breathing through a tube connected to an oxygen analyser, which measures the rate at which oxygen is being extracted from the inhaled air. The individual is subjected to a steadily increasing workload until he or she can continue no longer. Real-time display of oxygen uptake shows a linear increase with increasing workload until the maximal oxygen uptake is reached. At this point the graph levels off at what is known as the 'anaerobic threshold'. The exerciser is capable of a bit more effort, but very soon has to stop from exhaustion. Increasing oxygen uptake is facilitated by increasing heart rate, which follows a similar trajectory, increasing to its maximum at peak exercise.

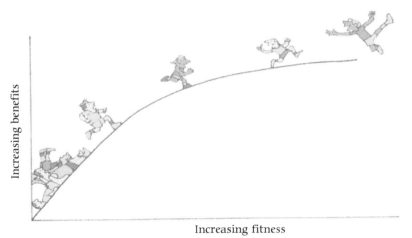

Relationship between exercise intensity and heart rate

Maximum oxygen uptake – VO_{2max} – is usually between 1.5 and 3.5 litres per minute. This is converted into millilitres per minute per kilogram of body weight by multiplying by 1,000 and dividing by the weight of the individual. It can be further converted into metabolic equivalents (METs) by dividing by 3.5, since a MET is 3.5ml/min/kg (see Chapter 3). So for a 70kg (11 stone) person with an oxygen uptake at maximum effort of 2 litres per minute:

$$VO_{2max} = 2,000\text{ml per minute}$$

and

2,000 divided by 70 gives the oxygen consumption in ml per minute per kg body weight = 28.6ml/min/kg

$$MET_{max} = 28.6 \text{ divided by } 3.5 = 8.16 \text{ METs}$$

Most measurements of fitness, however, estimate oxygen uptake by relying on the known oxygen cost of the exercise undertaken.

The motorised treadmill is the most popular method for use in the laboratory. A variety of different protocols can be used, the most popular being the famous Bruce protocol, devised by the Seattle-based cardiologist Robert Bruce. The treadmill is started at 1.7mph with a 10-degree slope and is increased every 3 minutes through seven stages to the maximum of 6.0mph and a 22-degree slope. The time spent on the treadmill before exhaustion can be used to predict VO_{2max}.

Bicycle ergometers are much more portable than treadmills and are the most popular instruments for use in 'field' studies. Estimation of exercise intensity requires the work done on the bicycle to be measured. Workload is controlled by the resistance to pedalling and speed of pedalling. With mechanically braked bicycles the resistance depends upon a weight applied to the braking system, and if workload is to be calculated the pedaller must cycle at a constant speed, using a metronome. For electronically braked machines the workload is set at the required level and resistance then varies with pedal speed, so a constant pedalling rate is not required. Workload is measured in watts (joules per second).

Again, a variety of protocols may be used. One such starts the individual at 25 or 50 or 75 watts and increases the workload by 25 watts every 3–5 minutes – long enough to reach 'steady-state' exercise. The cyclist continues to exhaustion and the oxygen uptake at this point is calculated from a knowledge of the oxygen cost of cycling.

Measuring your fitness for yourself

There are a number of benefits from being able to measure your own fitness:

- It can give you an idea of how fit – or unfit – you are in comparison with others of your own sex and age. You should be concerned if you find that you are average or less – most people are far less fit than they should be. You should not be content with anything less than 'above average'.

- Seeing just how unfit you are might (should) stimulate you to take up or increase exercise.

- It gives you a benchmark to measure future improvements and the effectiveness of whatever exercise you are taking.

The simplest rough indicator of physical fitness is your resting heart rate. For men any level above 70 and for women above 80 beats per minute may indicate reduced fitness. These levels work for large groups in identifying increased risk of cardiovascular disease and cancers,[2] but are too blunt a weapon for the individual.

There are several ways in which you can estimate your own VO_{2max} accurately enough to be useful. The best of these is the Cooper test, devised by Dr Kenneth Cooper from the US in the 1960s.[3] Anyone with the ability to walk unaided can do it – and here is how.

The Cooper test measures how far you can travel on foot in 12 minutes – as simple as that, yet it gives a remarkably accurate indicator of VO_{2max}. As you cover the distance, be aware of your limitations. Younger people and fitter older people can run for 12 minutes. If this is too hard for you, try a walk-jog, alternating fast walking with jogging. Older people and those who have not run for many years are best doing it at the fastest walk they can manage. Remember that 12 minutes of continuous exercise is longer than you might think. Don't start too fast.

There are several ways of measuring the distance:

1. If you have a smartphone, download a Cooper test app and just follow the instructions. The phone will measure the distance covered in 12 minutes, work out your VO_{2max} and tell you how you did. The app will also tell you how you compare with others of your age and gender. Misleadingly, it gives the same comparisons for everyone over the age of 60, so does not do justice to older folk (see below for a broader age spread of normal values).

2. If you have a GPS watch, use it to measure how far you have gone in 12 minutes.

3. Use a measured track (you can make this yourself on any reasonable-sized playing field) and note the distance around the track you can cover in 12 minutes.

The following table, which is adapted from Dr Cooper's findings, sets out the results from the distance covered in the 12 minutes, giving both your VO_{2max} and how you compare with everyone else of the same age and sex. Since Dr Cooper's figures stop at the age of 'over 60', I have added my age predictions for 70–79-year-olds and 80–89-year-olds. However, these predictions apply only to those who are able to complete 12 minutes of walking and this may not be the case for many older people. For them, the 6-minute walk test (see page 52) is a much better measure of their fitness and how it compares to the population at large.

After you have completed the test, you can compare your results to the norms and recommendations for your age and gender with the table opposite.

12-minute run/walk fitness-test results

Men

Age	Average (metres)	Average VO_{2max}
20–29	2200–2399m	40.1
30–39	1900–2299m	35.6
40–49	1700–2099m	31.2
50–59	1600–1999m	28.9
60–69	1400–1700m	23.4
70–79	1300–1600m	21.1
80–89	1100–1400m	18.0

Women

Age	Average (metres)	Average VO_{2max}
20–29	1800–2199m	33.4
30–39	1700–1999m	30.1
40–49	1500–1899m	26.7
50–59	1400–1699m	23.4
60–69	1300–1600m	21.1
70–79	1200–1500m	18.9
80–89	1100–1400m	17.8

To calculate your estimated VO_{2max} (in ml/min/kg) from the distance travelled in 12 minutes, use either of these formulas:

In miles: $VO_{2max} = (35.97 \times miles) - 11.29$

In kilometres: $VO_{2max} = (22.351 \times km) - 11.288$

For older, less fit people and those with heart or lung diseases, a 6-minute walk is often used and has also been shown to give an acceptable prediction of VO_{2max}. The procedure is much the same as the Cooper test but for 6 rather than 12 minutes and walking as fast as possible. Below is a table of expected results at different ages over 65. You will notice that the estimate of fitness given by this method is considerably lower than that given by the Cooper test. This is probably because the samples of individuals used to calculate the figures were rather different. I believe that the Cooper test sample population was considerably fitter than the majority of older people and I find the 6-minute walk test results more convincing.

6-minute walk fitness-test results

Men

Age	Average (metres)	Average VO_{2max}
65	596m	18.6
70	568m	18.0
75	534m	17.2
80	487m	16.3
85	427m	15.5
90	403m	14.2

Women

Age	Average (metres)	Average VO_{2max}
65	535m	17.3
70	510m	16.7
75	482m	16.0
80	443m	15.1
85	406m	14.3
90	358m	13.1

There are a lot of formulae for converting distance covered in the 6-minute test into VO_{2max} but none is very accurate. Some involve body mass index (BMI) and can be very complicated to work out. The best is this:

VO_{2max} in ml/min/kg = 0.023 multiplied by the 6-minute walk distance in metres plus 4.95

This works well for those whose maximum distance walked in 6 minutes is 600 metres or less, but underestimates VO_{2max} for those who can go further. For them, the Cooper test is more accurate.

* * *

The figures I have given for average fitness at different ages must be taken with more than a pinch of salt. The average fitness level and the variation in fitness differ from one group to another. There have been many studies to try to determine the average fitness of the population as a whole, with variations from very unfit to very fit – but the results such surveys have produced show wide discrepancies because of the way in which the subjects have been selected and the nature of the testing systems used. In some cases the figures are derived from people who have volunteered to be tested; in other cases the sample is drawn from a particular set, such as those seeking routine health checks; and in a few cases the individuals being tested have been chosen randomly.[4] Even for the most representative group tested, the average level of fitness will exceed reality because there will be a proportion of the subjects who have physical problems that prevent them completing the test. Their results are therefore discounted, thus raising the average. Given that population measurements apply only to those members of the population who can complete the test and the proportion who are unable to do this increases with age, the overestimate of population fitness levels is much greater for older age groups.

The difficulty in giving the normal range of physical fitness in the general population is illustrated by the two best and most representative investigations carried out in England over the past 30 years:

- **The Allied Dunbar Fitness Survey** in 1990 tested a sample of 1,741 adults aged 16–74 chosen at random in 30 locations around the UK. They used a treadmill in a central mobile laboratory. For men, the average VO_{2max} fell from 55.5 in the 16–34 age group to 32 in the 65–74 age group.

- **The Health Survey for England** in 2008[5] also tested a random sample – 1,969 people – using a step test in the individuals' homes. For men, the average VO_{2max} fell from 40.9 in the 16–34 age group to 29.9 in the 65–74 group.

It would be expected that both studies should produce comparable results, but in practice the earlier study suggested that in 1990 the population of England was significantly fitter than it was in 2008. There are several explanations for such a disparity: perhaps the samples were in some way biased differently; the testing methods were not comparable; it was easier to get the subjects to exercise harder in a laboratory than in their own homes where emergency help was less available; or maybe we really are getting steadily less fit, the victims of our increasingly sedentary lifestyles.

All this explains why any table of normal fitness levels must be flawed. However, I do believe that it can be helpful to know roughly where you fit into the range of possible fitness levels, so I have constructed the tables on page 56 for this purpose. The figures have been compiled from a number of sources to give the best guesses for each age and sex.[4-9] They are only a guide, but should give you an idea of where you fit into the scheme of things.

Two additional points. Firstly, after the mid-twenties physical fitness declines throughout life – by about 0.5 per cent per annum in early adult life but getting steeper in middle age at about 1 per cent each year and accelerating in old age to about 2 per cent or more each year. This has been clearly demonstrated in a survey known as the FIT study of nearly 70,000 US citizens.[10]

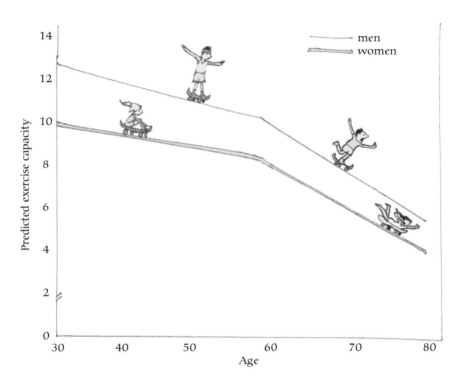

Predicted fitness levels in METs at different ages in men and women

Taking moderate exercise does not change this rate of decline, but it does of course still give a better fitness level at any age than being less active.[11] More vigorous training, however, as in older athletes, does decrease the rate of decline – to about 0.5 per cent each year even in old age.[12,13]

At any age women are significantly less fit than men, mostly because they have a different body composition with a greater fat content. When this is allowed for by adjusting the figure for fat-free mass, there is little difference between the sexes.

Range of VO$_{2max}$ for men

Age	Poor	Below average	Average	Good	Very good
20–29	<35	35–38	38–45	45–50	>50
30–39	<31	31–35	35–41	41–49	>49
40–49	<30	30–33	33–39	39–48	>48
50–59	<26	26–31	31–36	36–45	>45
60–69	<21	21–29	29–33	33–41	>41
70–79	<15	15–25	25–29	29–36	>36

Range of VO$_{2max}$ for women

Age	Poor	Below average	Average	Good	Very good
20–29	<23	23–33	29–33	33–41	>41
30–39	<23	23–27	27–31	31–40	>40
40–49	<21	21–24	24–29	29–37	>37
50–59	<20	20–23	23–27	27–35	>35
60–69	<18	18–21	21–25	25–31	>31
70–79	<12	12–19	19–21	21–28	>28

– **6**–

How Often, How Hard and How Long?

If you still look cute after your workout – you didn't train hard enough.
Anon.

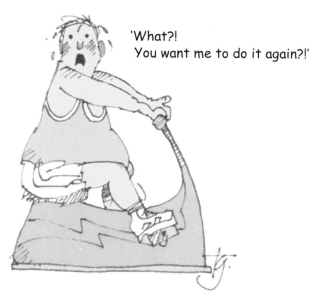

'What?!
You want me to do it again?!'

Here is a quick guide that is more or less applicable to any endurance exercise. The following graphs indicate the frequency, intensity and duration needed to increase your aerobic capacity – i.e. your physical fitness. These are sometimes known as the FITT principles – Frequency, Intensity, Time, Type of exercise.

Frequency – how often?

This graph shows the relationship between exercise frequency and increase in fitness as measured by VO_{2max}.

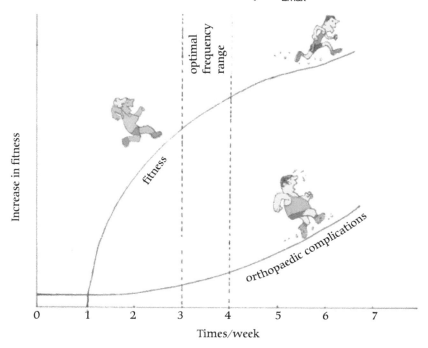

How Often: Exercise frequency v. increase in fitness

Exercising once a week has little effect, twice weekly a moderate effect, three or four times weekly a better effect, but after that there is a fall-off in the benefit of more frequent training. In addition, the more often you train, the greater the risk of sprains and strains to your joints and muscles.

Intensity – how hard?

This graph shows the relationship between intensity of exercise (as measured as the percentage of maximum heart rate reached) and increase in fitness as measured by VO_{2max}.

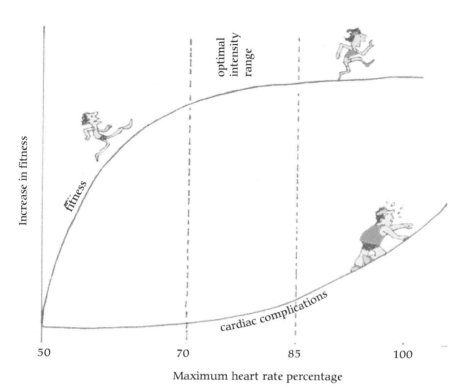

How Hard: Exercise intensity v. increase in fitness

Again, increasing effort brings increasing rewards, but there is a point beyond which there is a reducing return. This point is reached at between roughly 70 and 85 per cent maximum heart rate. For people with heart disease, exercising to very high heart rates brings an increased danger of complications, particularly disturbances of rhythm.

Just a word about heart rate. As I said on page 33, predicted maximum heart rate (PMHR) is about 220 minus your age. So 70 per cent of PMHR is about 170 minus your age and 85 per cent PMHR is about 195 minus your age. When you are exercising at between 70 and 85 per cent PMHR, you can just about talk with someone with you – you should be comfortably short of breath but not gasping. If you are taking any medication that might slow heart rate (particularly beta-blockers and some calcium channel blockers) these figures do not apply. You must rely on how hard it feels to exercise – see Borg scale or RPE opposite.

Time – how long?

This graph shows the relationship between duration of exercise sessions and increase in fitness as measured by VO_{2max}.

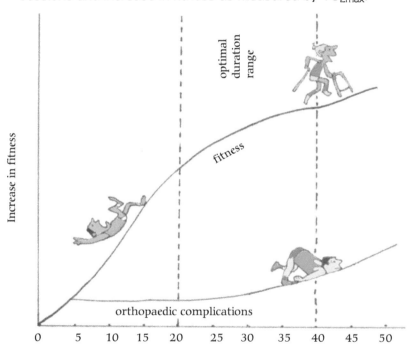

How Long: Exercise duration v. increase in fitness

There is a steady increase in physical fitness for increase in duration of exercise up to about 30–40 minutes, but after that there is a flattening of the curve, with less and less benefit the greater the time spent training. Again, the more time you spend training, the greater the risk of musculoskeletal injury.

The total amount of dynamic aerobic activity can be expressed as 'exercise volume', which is the product of average METs multiplied by the time involved in minutes. It has been suggested that the goal for maintaining good health should be between 500 and 1,000 MET minutes per week. Take the example of walking at, say, 3.5mph. This uses about 6.4 METs, so the target would take between 1 hour 18 minutes (499 MET minutes) and 2 hours 36 minutes (998 MET minutes) of walking per week. If you are stepping out faster at, say, 4mph (7.1 METs), the goal is reached with between 1 hour 10 minutes and 2 hours 20 minutes of walking per week.

Type of exercise

I have described the first three elements of the FITT – Frequency, Intensity and Time – but not the final T, the Type of exercise. I do have a bit to say about this, scattered throughout, but it is not one of the remits of this book. I am very keen that anyone reading the book – and anyone not reading it – should increase their physical activity, but I am reluctant to make any particular recommendations about what type of exercise you should do. Just do what you will enjoy; it is doing you the most good if you enjoy it and it makes you short of breath. If your chosen activity satisfies these two criteria you can only benefit. There is little evidence that what you have chosen is better or worse than any other form of exercise.

Rate of perceived exertion (RPE)

It is not easy to measure your own heart rate – as soon as you stop to feel your pulse, your heart rate slows. Pulse-rate monitors can do it for you, but many people prefer to rely simply on how hard the exercise feels to them. This is best done using the RPE, devised by a Danish physiologist called Gunnar Borg and often referred to as the Borg scale. It is expressed (overleaf) as a score from 0 to 10 which describes how hard you are finding the exercise.

0	none
0.5	very, very light
1	very light
2	light
3	moderate
4	somewhat heavy
5	heavy
6	–
7	very heavy
8	–
9	very, very heavy
10	–

Predicted maximum heart rate usually reaches the 70–85 per cent level at between numbers 4 and 6 on the scale.

So how much exercise should you take?

The effectiveness of exercise is proportional to its intensity and total dose. From the above, you would be right to presume that optimal exercising should be about 30 to 40 minutes of exercise three or four times per week to a level that makes you reasonably out of breath. This is also sufficient exercise to have a highly significant effect on both the prevention and treatment of a number of diseases. It is not enough exercise if you wish to compete as a serious sportsman. Committed runners, cyclists, squash players, footballers and competitive tennis players, for instance, need to be far fitter than would be allowed by this relatively modest regime – but they do risk injury for their sport and the older they become the bigger a problem this is.

The current NHS guideline recommends a mix of aerobic exercise and muscle strengthening.

To stay healthy, adults aged 19–64 should try to be active daily and should do:

- At least 150 minutes (2 hours and 30 minutes) of moderate-intensity aerobic activity such as cycling or fast walking every week, **and**

- muscle-strengthening activities on 2 or more days a week that work all major muscle groups (legs, hips, back, abdomen, chest, shoulders and arms).

OR

- 75 minutes (1 hour and 15 minutes) of vigorous-intensity aerobic activity such as running or a game of singles tennis every week, **and**

- muscle-strengthening activities on 2 or more days a week that work all major muscle groups (legs, hips, back, abdomen, chest, shoulders and arms).

OR

- An equivalent mix of moderate- and vigorous-intensity aerobic activity every week (for example two 30-minute runs plus 30 minutes of fast walking), **and**

- muscle-strengthening activities on 2 or more days a week that work all major muscle groups (legs, hips, back, abdomen, chest, shoulders and arms).

A rule of thumb is that 1 minute of vigorous-intensity activity is about the same as 2 minutes of moderate-intensity activity.

One way to do your recommended 150 minutes of weekly physical activity is to do 30 minutes on 5 days a week.

Examples of activities that require moderate effort for most people include:

- walking fast
- water aerobics
- riding a bike on level ground or with few hills
- doubles tennis
- pushing a lawn mower
- hiking
- skateboarding
- rollerblading
- volleyball
- basketball

Moderate-intensity activity will raise your heart rate and make you breathe faster and feel warmer. One way to tell if you're working at a moderate intensity is if you can still talk, but you can't sing the words to a song.

What counts as vigorous-intensity activity?

There is substantial evidence that vigorous-intensity activity can bring health benefits over and above that of moderate-intensity activity. Examples of activities that require vigorous effort for most people include:

- jogging or running
- swimming fast
- riding a bike fast or on hills
- singles tennis
- football
- rugby
- rope skipping
- hockey
- aerobics
- gymnastics
- martial arts

Vigorous-intensity activity means that you're breathing hard and fast, and your heart rate has gone up quite a bit. If you're working at this level, you won't be able to say more than a few words without pausing for a breath.

In general, 75 minutes of vigorous-intensity activity can give similar health benefits to 150 minutes of moderate-intensity activity.

What counts as muscle-strengthening activity?

Muscle strength is necessary for daily activities, to build and maintain strong bones, to regulate blood sugar and blood pressure and to help maintain a healthy weight.

Muscle-strengthening exercises are counted in repetitions and sets. A repetition is 1 complete movement of an activity, like lifting a weight or doing a sit-up. A set is a group of repetitions.

For each activity, try to do 8–12 repetitions in each set. Try to do at least 1 set of each muscle-strengthening activity. You'll get even more benefits if you do 2 or 3 sets.[1]

These are some examples of muscle-strengthening activities. They include types of exercise which are also counted in the 'moderate' and 'vigorous' categories above:

- lifting weights
- using resistance bands
- heavy gardening (think fork and spade work or pushing the lawn mower)
- stair-climbing, particularly carrying the shopping or the vacuum cleaner
- hill-walking
- cycling, particularly on hills
- dancing, particularly if you have to lift your partner
- press-ups
- sit-ups
- squats

How good are these recommendations?

They are both realistic and highly beneficial. Although this recommended level of aerobic exercise is considerably less than the optimal dose I have described above, it is still enough to bring an appreciable increase in physical fitness together with health and longevity benefits. Note, however, that the NHS guidelines do point out that there is substantial evidence that more vigorous-intensity activity can bring health benefits over and above that of moderate-intensity activity. See below for the comparative effects of moderate-intensity and more vigorous exercise on lifespan, etc.

Almost identical recommended exercise guidelines have been produced by a number of countries and continental groups. There is no science to these recommendations, which are a compromise between what is ideal and what is achievable. The recommended level has been plucked from the sky and has no real evidence to support it. The benefits of exercise increase with increasing exercise level, but the more exercise that is recommended the smaller the chance of its being taken up. No one has yet demonstrated the crossover point beyond which the benefit of exercise at a population level is cancelled out by the reduction in uptake! In 2018 the 'Physical activity guidelines for health and prosperity in the United States' were published.[2] The overall levels of recommended activity were not changed from previous guidelines, but the way in which the exercise was broken up was different: 'Even short-duration activity lasting less than 10 minutes is beneficial.'

One more wrinkle – as we get older the benefits of exercise get greater and greater but we take less and less of it. One study has used US figures to calculate that average walking time for 20–29-year-olds is about 30 minutes per day, falling to about 9 minutes per day by the age of 70–79.[3] Very reasonably, they argue that it is futile to advise the elderly to triple their exercise – they just won't do it. The target for everyone should not be a fixed amount of exercise but an increase that is within the bounds of possible attainment. They also give reference to the

UK Chief Medical Officer's statement: 'the majority of UK older adults have low levels of activity so it is important to emphasise that they can achieve some benefits from increasing their activity even if it is below the recommendation'. Indeed, the greatest relative benefit is achieved by increasing from doing nothing to doing something, even if that something is not very much.

Even the somewhat modest levels of exercise recommended by the NHS are nowhere near being met by the vast majority of UK citizens, as we will see in the next chapter.

– 7 –

How Much Exercise Do We *Really* Take?

Take care of your body. It's the only place you have to live.

Jim Rohn

There are a number of answers to this question, depending upon who is making the estimate and how they have measured it. Some of the regular surveys that assess physical activity in the population include the Health Survey for England (HSE),[1] the Active People Survey,[2] the National Travel Survey[3] and the General Household Survey.[4]

The HSE compares current population activity with the Department of Health recommendations: these have changed subtly over the years and the current guidelines are given in the previous chapter (pages 63–5). The HSE uses validated questionnaires completed by wide sections of the population to assess the level of compliance with these guidelines. Different types of activity are summarised into a frequency–duration scale which takes into account the time spent participating in physical activities and the number of active days in the last week. By this measure the proportion of adults meeting the recommendation has increased steadily since 1997 for men and 1998 for women. In 1997, 32 per cent of men met the recommendation, increasing to 43 per cent in 2012. Among women, 21 per cent met the recommendation in 1998, increasing to 32 per cent in 2012.

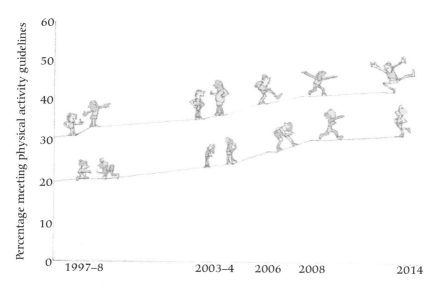

Increase over time of self-reported compliance with exercise guidelines

After 2012 the recommendations changed to include shorter bursts of activity, so the figures for the past few years cannot be compared with the earlier figures. Currently the estimates are that 66 per cent of men and 58 per cent of women meet the guidelines. Be aware, however, that these results depend upon the accuracy of the self-assessment of the individuals completing the questionnaires and are likely to be substantial overestimates – see below.

The 2008 HSE report found that, based on the participants' self-reported data, 39 per cent of men and 29 per cent of women in the whole survey met the exercise recommendations of the Chief Medical Officer (CMO). Increasing age and increasing BMI were associated with decreasing levels of activity. At age 16–24, 52 per cent of men and 35 per cent of women met the recommendations. The numbers fell steadily over the next three decades of life to 41 per cent and 31 per cent. Thereafter the fall was more precipitate, to 9 per cent and 6 per cent for the over-75s.

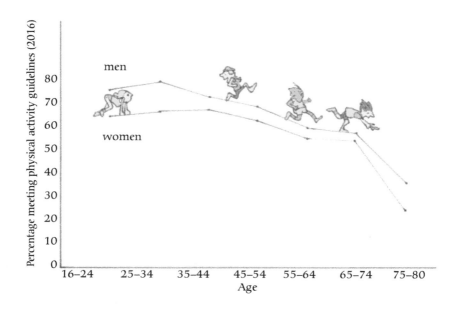

Relationship between age and self-assessed exercise guideline compliance

Like other HSE surveys, the report gives a huge amount of additional data, including the effect of obesity and social status on activity and also the different activities included in different age and sex groupings.

In 2011 the Department of Health modified its recommendations, as explained in the previous chapter: 'Adults should aim to be active daily. Over a week, activity should add up to at least 150 minutes (2½ hours) of moderate-intensity activity in bouts of 10 minutes or more – one way to approach this is to do 30 minutes on at least five days a week. Alternatively, comparable benefits can be achieved through 75 minutes of vigorous-intensity activity spread across the week or a combination of moderate- and vigorous-intensity activity.'[5] The recommendations also added muscle-strengthening activities on two or more days per week that work all major muscle groups (legs, hips, back, abdomen, chest, shoulders and arms).

Using the new guidelines, the HSE 2012 estimated that 34 per cent of men and 24 per cent of women aged 16 and over met their recommendations. In both sexes, the proportion who met the guidelines generally decreased with age, reduced household income and increased BMI.[6] Compared with the 2008 survey, there was an increase in those meeting the recommendation for aerobic activity. Considering just the aerobic exercise component, the numbers reaching the targets in 2012 were 67 per cent of men and 55 per cent of women, and by 2016 this had reduced to 66 per cent for men and increased to 58 per cent for women.[7] So it does seem that we are improving a bit in our exercise habit – or getting better at self-deception.

I have given greater details of the HSE 2008 report because that year the survey added a separate assessment of activity levels – it actually *measured* what people did. The comparison with what they *said* they did is startling. Questionnaire estimates of activity levels rely entirely on self-reporting. However, people are born liars and the human tendency is to exaggerate both to ourselves and, perhaps even more, to others the amount of good stuff we do. This has been termed 'social desirability bias'! The unreliability of self-reported activity is nicely confirmed by the added information sought by the HSE 2008 survey. They used accelerometers (a sort of sophisticated pedometer) to record the frequency, intensity and duration of physical activity in one-minute 'epochs', showing accurately the actual daily activity of their subjects over a period of one week. Based on the results of the accelerometer study, 6 per cent of men and 4 per cent of women achieved the government's recommended physical activity level – just 15 per cent of the level of compliance indicated by individuals' own questionnaire responses – revealing a staggering level of either self-deception or just downright lying! Men and women aged 16–34 were most likely to reach the recommended physical activity level (11 per cent and 8 per cent respectively), while the proportion of both men and women meeting the recommendations fell in the older age groups. On average, men spent 31 minutes in moderate or vigorous activity

(MVPA) in total per day and women an average of 24 minutes. However, most of this was sporadic activity, and only about a third of it was accrued in the bouts of 10 minutes or longer that count towards the government recommendations.

When the effects of physical fitness are compared with stated activity levels, it is physical fitness that is a far better predictor of future heart disease and mortality, particularly in younger subjects.[8] Hardly surprising, is it? Our fitness level is an excellent reflection of how much exercise we actually take as compared with what we might like to think we take.

So just how fit are we? The answer can be found in the next chapter.

– 8 –
So Just How Fit Are We?

Any casual observer can tell at a glance I'm not the person I think I am.
Marty Rubin, writer and humorist

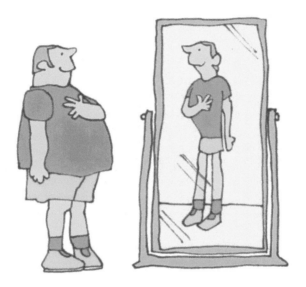

The answer to the question posed by the title of this chapter is: a lot less than we should be and a lot, *lot* less than we think we are.

The first attempt to assess the nation's physical fitness was published in 1990 – the Allied Dunbar National Fitness Survey (ADNFS).[1] This was conducted in a representative sample of English adults aged 16–96 years between February and November 1990. A total of 4,316 participants (76 per cent response rate) were interviewed about a range of sociodemographic characteristics and lifestyle factors, such as diet, physical activity (type, frequency and duration), smoking, alcohol, sleep, stress and social support. A sub-sample of 2,767 participants also underwent a physical appraisal, which included objective assessment of body dimension, composition, flexibility, and cardiorespiratory and muscular fitness. The findings were shocking. More than 7 out of 10 men and 8 out of 10 women fell below their age-appropriate activity level for achieving a health benefit. About 1 in 6 had done no activity for 20 minutes or more in the past month. The level of inactivity increased with age: 10 per cent of 16–20-year-olds took no exercise, increasing to 40 per cent of 65–74-year-olds. When tested on a treadmill, the proportion of men unable to sustain uphill walking at 3mph rose from 4 per cent in the 16–24-year-olds to 81 per cent in the 65–74 year group. For women, the equivalent proportions were 34 per cent and 92 per cent. The figures for muscle strength were no more encouraging, 50 per cent of women over 55 being unable to walk upstairs without assistance. Interestingly, though fitness tended to decline with age, many older individuals were as fit as or fitter than some of the much younger subjects. Astonishingly, 80 per cent of both men and women of all ages incorrectly believed that they did enough exercise to keep fit – yet more evidence of the human's capacity for self-deception.

The HSE 2008 is the best source of information on the measured cardiovascular fitness of a representative sample of the UK population.[2] Adults aged 16–74 underwent a step test – stepping up and down a single step of determined height at a fixed rate for a maximum of 8 minutes. The pace of stepping increased throughout the test. Heart-rate measurements were taken during and after the test, then combined with the resting heart rate to provide an estimate of the individual's maximal oxygen uptake (VO_{2max}).The information in the HSE 2008 was analysed to allow comparisons to be made between the HSE 2008 and the ADNFS, which involved converting the results of the step test from the HSE to indicate the percentage of adults who could sustain walking at 3mph on the flat and on a 5 per cent incline. Key findings from the HSE 2008 were:

• Men had higher cardiovascular fitness levels than women, with an average level of VO_{2max} of 36.3ml/min/kg for men and 32.0ml/min/kg for women. In both sexes, the mean VO_{2max} decreased with age.

• Cardiovascular fitness was lower on average among those who were obese (32.3ml/min/kg among men and 28.1ml/min/kg among women) than among those who were neither overweight nor obese (38.8ml/min/kg and 33.9ml/min/kg respectively).

• Virtually all participants were deemed able to walk at 3mph on the flat but 84 per cent of men and 97 per cent of women would require moderate exertion for this activity. However, 32 per cent of men and 60 per cent of women were not fit enough to sustain walking at 3mph up a 5 per cent incline. Lack of fitness increased with age.

• Physical fitness was compared to self-reported physical activity. Average VO_{2max} decreased, and the proportion classified as unfit increased as self-reported physical activity level decreased.

There have been a number of other studies of physical fitness in the 'population', but the HSE figures are probably the most meaningful in the real world because they deliberately included as broad a cross-section of society as possible. Longitudinal studies, which examine the same people over a number of years, give more accurate estimates of the effects of age than cross-sectional samples, which examine all the subjects at one point in time.

Although HSE annual surveys indicate that more of us are complying with the government's exhortations to reach their exercise targets, there is evidence that this is not always translating into increased levels of fitness. For instance, the number of British military reservists failing their fitness assessments increased from 20 per cent in 2015 to 29 per cent in 2018.

– 9 –
Evidence: Interpreting the Science

The fact that an opinion has been widely held is no evidence whatever that it is not utterly absurd. Bertrand Russell

The heart of this book is the effect of exercise (or lack of it) on health and disease, and the extent to which exercise can both prevent a number of diseases and also contribute to their treatment. But I am not going to expect you to take me at my word – I will be presenting evidence for what I tell you. So I must start by saying a few words about evidence as applied to facts and beliefs in the medical setting. In the case of exercise and health, we will be talking about cause and effect.

When it comes to exercise as a factor in health and disease, an important source of evidence is found in epidemiology – sorry, there I go again with long words. 'Epidemiology is the study and analysis of the patterns, causes, and effects of health and disease conditions in defined populations. It is the cornerstone of public health, and shapes policy decisions and evidence-based practice by identifying risk factors for disease and targets for preventive healthcare'.[1] OK, that's pretty indigestible. In simple terms, epidemiology is the observation of associations between disease and certain behaviours, environmental conditions and physical states. For example, when Professors Richard Doll and Tim Peto from Oxford identified cigarettes as the main cause of lung cancer, they used epidemiological evidence – the observation that people who smoked cigarettes had a far higher incidence of lung cancer than those who did not. A lot of the evidence related to the effects of exercise are epidemiologically based, for instance the finding that people who take a lot of exercise are less likely to develop type 2 diabetes.

Both these examples demonstrate only associations, not proof of cause. Association is not the same as causation – though it may be! Take this example: during the period in the 20th century when the incidence of coronary disease was increasing rapidly, so was the use of the radio – but few people believe that coronary disease is caused by radio waves. In the case of smoking and lung cancer, however, there is no other reasonable explanation and there are good biological reasons to believe that smoking might cause lung disease. In the case of exercise and diabetes, we cannot be quite so sure. There may be other 'confounders' – that is to say, other factors with which both exercise and diabetes are associated, such as sugar consumption. If exercisers consume less sugar than non-exercisers, that might be the explanation for the association. There are many differences between exercisers and non-exercisers and it would be impossible to find groups of each whose other characteristics were identical, so many of the associations that I will describe below are just that – associations with a very strong presumption of a causal link.

Stronger evidence of causation is provided by the clinical trial. The purest form is the randomised, double-blind, controlled trial (RCT). This is best understood in the example of a drug trial. A group of individuals with a particular condition is selected to clarify the effect of the drug and they are divided randomly into two groups. One group receives the treatment and the other (the control group) receives a placebo – that is, an inert pill that looks the same as the real treatment. Neither the person giving the treatment and assessing its effect nor the patient receiving it knows who is getting the real treatment and who is getting the placebo. At the end of a predefined period the code is broken and the difference between the two groups analysed. If a trial of a cancer treatment is being tested, this might be the cure rate, and if the cure rate is significantly higher in the treatment group than in the control group it can be inferred that the drug is effective. There are lots of possible pitfalls even in this very straightforward scenario. The patients might not have complied properly with the treatment – this is most likely for the treatment group if the drug has unpleasant side effects. The randomisation process might not be perfect. Despite the randomisation, there may be unexpected differences between the two groups. The statistical analysis has its own problems. In clinical trials statistical significance is reached if the chance of the difference found between the two groups is less than 1 in 20 (in statistical shorthand, $p = <0.05$). With a clearly effective treatment this can be derived from a trial with small numbers of patients. The less obvious the effect, the more patients will be needed in the trial to show it. The more patients needed in the trial to show an effective outcome, the less effective the drug must be. If the number needed is very great, a statistically significant effect might be clinically *in*significant – not worth the candle. The counterside to this is that small trials are more likely to produce erroneous results – the bigger the trial, the more reliable a test it is. Even apparently well-conducted RCTs can yield results with problems of interpretation. When such trials are carried out by pharmaceutical firms on their own products, they are far more likely to have a positive outcome than independently funded and conducted trials (see page 80).

If you think that all that is bad enough, just consider the difficulties of carrying out randomised, controlled trials of exercise! For a start, they cannot be double-blind – treatment group members know they are in the treatment group and it is quite hard to prevent the observers from knowing too. Compliance can be a nightmare and there may be cross-contamination – that is, members of the control group may start exercising, even if they have been asked not to. When I carried out a randomised, controlled, but not blinded, trial of exercise for patients following heart attacks, one of the non-exercise *controls* bought himself a static bicycle on his way home from his initial exercise test!

A further difficulty in most epidemiologic studies and in many trials of exercise is that the estimated amount of physical activity depends on the evidence of the individual. Unfortunately this is highly unreliable, as we saw in Chapter 8, since most people greatly overestimate how much exercise they take. An alternative measure is the physical fitness of the person involved. This is independent of the lies told by the subject, both to the researcher and to himself, so should be a much more reliable measure – and almost certainly it is. However, fitness level is not wholly determined by the amount of exercise you take: there is also a genetic component, and this reduces the accuracy of fitness level as a reflection of exercise-taking.

There is one more level of evidence which in some instances can provide the strongest evidence – the systematic review and meta-analysis. These are most useful when the numbers required to show an effect in an RCT are larger than can be reasonably recruited in a single trial. It is also an essential technique for unravelling the facts when different studies of the same topic come up with different answers. A systematic review answers a defined research question by collecting and summarising all the evidence collected through observation that fits pre-specified eligibility criteria. A meta-analysis uses statistical methods to summarise the results of these studies. In other words, a meta-analysis is a summation of the results of all the trials carried out using the particular intervention under investigation. The total number of subjects is much larger than in single trials and the results should therefore be that much more convincing. Again, there are problems. Different trials are different in many aspects and combining them sometimes involves mixing oranges and pears. The choice of trials for inclusion is crucial if a particular question is to be answered – there must be as many similarities as possible. And there is the ever-present bias of the tendency to publish trials with a positive outcome but not those with a negative outcome.

Medicine is very far from being a perfect science – it is said that half of what doctors believe to be true today will, in time, be shown to be wrong. The trouble is that we do not know which half! Interpreting evidence is a huge problem, but it is at the heart of 'evidence-based medicine'. This book does not attempt to give a full systematic review of all the evidence for each statement on the effects of exercise, but I will include some of the more important or convincing research. In particular, I will be referring frequently to 'Cochrane Reviews'. The Cochrane Collaboration is an independent non-profit group that conducts systematic reviews and meta-analyses of RCTs of healthcare interventions across all aspects of medical treatments. If you need or wish to check on the evidence for any particular treatment, just Google 'Cochrane' and enter their website for the most comprehensive assessment of evidence-based interventions or drugs in the world. Helpfully, they include a layman's summary of the evidence and what it means.

Presentation of evidence

It is very easy to be misled by the way in which evidence is presented. Those with an axe to grind, including those funding the study, tend to present their results in the way that is most likely to persuade the reader that the treatment is effective. Also, negative studies are much less likely to reach the light of day than those with positive findings. This is particularly likely to bias the published results of drug trials.[1]

Fortunately, exercise studies are seldom sponsored by commercial organisations, but nevertheless the authors of such studies do sometimes have an interest in the outcomes – be aware of this possible bias.

One more point on the presentation of evidence. The benefit of a particular intervention is usually expressed in terms of change in risk and may be presented as a change in *relative* risk or a change in *absolute* risk. A change in relative risk usually makes the treatment seem much more attractive than a change in absolute risk.

- **Absolute risk** of a disease is the risk of developing the disease over a period of time and may be expressed as a fraction – say, 1 in 20; as a percentage – in this case 5 per cent; or as a decimal – in this case 0.05.

- **Relative risk** is used to compare the risk in two different groups of people. For example, the groups could be smokers and non-smokers. All sorts of groups are compared to others in medical research to see if belonging to a particular group increases or decreases your risk of developing certain diseases. For instance, research has shown that smokers have a higher risk of developing heart disease compared to (relative to) non-smokers.

Let us say that the absolute risk of developing heart disease is 4 in 100 (4 per cent) in non-smokers, but the relative risk of the disease is increased by 50 per cent in smokers. The 50 per cent relates to the 4 – so the absolute increase in the risk is 50 per cent of 4, which is 2. So, the absolute risk of smokers developing this disease is 6 in 100. If the two groups are compared, the increase in risk brought about by smoking is 2 in 100 – for every 100 smokers, 2 more individuals will develop heart disease compared to non-smokers.

When comparing the results of treatments, whether the outcomes are expressed as absolute or relative improvements can have a big effect on how good the treatment looks. The less common the condition, the truer this is. Look at the example of the risk of a heart attack and how this can be reduced by taking a particular drug. The risk of a heart attack over the next 10 years in a group of women aged between 40 and 50 may be, say, 1 in 100 – 1 per cent. If taking the drug in question reduces the risk to 1 in 200 (0.5 per cent) it may be reported that the risk of a heart attack, the relative risk, was halved in this group. However, the absolute risk is a reduction from two deaths to one death for every 200 women – an absolute reduction of 1 in 200. In other words, 200 women would have to take the drug for 10 years to prevent one new heart attack – which seems rather less impressive than halving the risk. Sometimes the effectiveness of a treatment is then expressed as 'number needed to treat', i.e. the number of people who need to take the treatment for just one person to benefit – in this case 200.

Mortality

Mortality rates are often used as outcome measures to compare the efficacy of different drugs and other treatments. Since the ultimate mortality for any treatment regime is 100 per cent – we all die in the end – 'mortality' when used for this end has to be qualified. There are two ways of doing this:

1. Mortality is expressed as the death rate over the period of study and compared between the groups being studied.

2. The death rate of the group being studied is compared with the known death rate of the whole population of the same age and gender – it is usually expressed as deaths per 1,000 persons per year.

Interpreting the evidence

So, facts unsupported by evidence should be questioned. Even when evidence seems to support the facts you must be alert to the possibilities of error. Very little evidence is unarguable – but it is a great deal better than any other way of reaching the truth, about exercise as about anything else.

– 10 –

Exercise, Fitness and Disease: How They All Relate

Better to hunt in fields, for health unbought,
Than fee the doctor for a nauseous draught.
The wise, for cure, on exercise depend;
God never made his work for man to mend.
John Dryden, 1700

There are many excellent and commendable reasons for being a regular exerciser. Firstly, it is or should be fun. If it is not, find a different exercise or sport. Failing that, find the exercise that you dislike least – it will still be a small investment for a massive dividend.

Regular exercise makes you feel good – even smug! Everything is easier to do, and you can do so much more than the couch potato. It can be an excellent vehicle for social activities. Most of all, it gives you a longer, more enjoyable and illness-free life.

This chapter discusses the different diseases and conditions to which man is heir and which are influenced by exercise, physical fitness and physical training. I will start with some of the risk factors for disease. Most chronic diseases – non-communicable diseases (NCDs) – do not have a single simple cause but a variety of contributory risk factors which come together to make you ill. Most of these are lifestyle choices. It is often difficult to decide whether a particular condition is a risk factor or a disease, particularly since many diseases are also risk factors for other diseases. So in the pages that follow I will simply discuss risk factors and diseases without trying to distinguish between them. What you will find is the close interconnectedness between the different risk factors and different diseases – mainly the degenerative diseases of middle and later life – and the fact that regular exercise not only prevents these diseases but is also an effective treatment for most of them.

Obesity

A bear, however hard he tries, grows tubby without exercise.
A. A. Milne

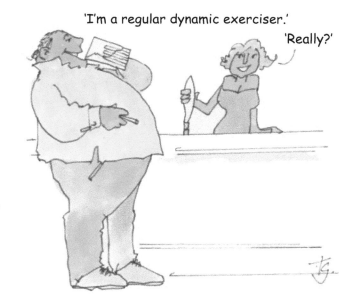

The standard way of measuring weight compared with height is body mass index (BMI), which is weight in kilograms divided by height in metres squared. So a 70kg (about 11 stone) person who is 1.75m (about 5 foot 9 inches) tall has a BMI of 70 divided by 1.75 squared, which is 70 divided by 3.0625, which comes to about 22.9. You do not need to work out your own BMI so laboriously. Just Google 'BMI' and there are plenty of websites that will work it out for you using either pounds and feet or kilograms and centimetres.

The ideal BMI is generally accepted as between 18.5 and 25. Between 25 and 30 is 'overweight', between 30 and 40 is 'obese' and over 40 is 'morbidly obese'. For the purposes of longevity, a BMI between 20 and 25 is optimal.[1] Weights higher than this carry an increasing risk of coronary disease and type 2 diabetes, of which much more later.

However, there is more to weight than BMI. It also matters where you store your excess fat. Obesity can be predominantly either central or peripheral. Those with central obesity store fat in the abdominal cavity and have paunches or beer bellies – the apple shape. Those with peripheral obesity store it on their hips, bums and thighs – the pear shape. Being an apple is much more dangerous than being a pear. So when it comes to assessing risk

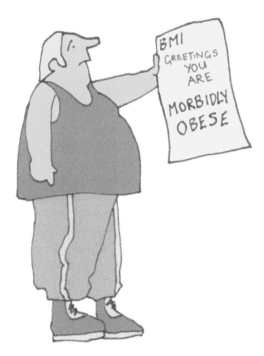

from obesity, mainly risk for cardiovascular diseases and premature death, waist measurement seems to give a better picture than BMI. The upper limit of recommended waist size for men is 102cm (40 inches) and for women 88cm (35 inches). With higher measurements, the risk for cardiovascular disease (CVD), diabetes and high blood pressure all rise steeply. An alternative parameter is the waist/hip ratio (waist circumference divided by hip circumference). For men this should be below 1.0 and for women below 0.8.

Obesity is not a new condition. One of the oldest surviving human carvings, the Venus of Willendorf, created some 27,000 years ago, depicts a strikingly obese woman.

Hippocrates, in about 500 BC, reported that obese people were at increased risk of sudden death. More recently, in

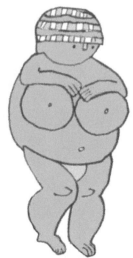

The Willendorf Venus

1727, a British physician named Thomas Short wrote, 'No age has seen more instances of corpulency than our own'.[2] To which the proper response might be, 'Man, you ain't seen nothin' yet!' Obesity is a huge and growing problem in most Western countries and the figures published about its extent are as gross as the problem itself. The weight of the average person in the UK has risen by more than 1.5kg (3 lb) every decade since 1970. The horrifying statistics go on and on. The UK is the most overweight nation in Western Europe and our levels of obesity are growing even faster than those of the US.

The seeds of obesity are sown in childhood. In Reception year (aged 4–5) 9.5 per cent of children are obese and by Year 6 (aged 10–11) this has increased to 19 per cent and is still rising. The rate of severe obesity has grown from 3.2 per cent to 4 per cent in the last decade and the inexorable increase in childhood obesity is behind the very serious problem of rising levels of childhood type 2 diabetes (see page 105). Government initiatives to reduce childhood obesity have failed miserably and interventions in schools have also mostly been unsuccessful. This may not be unrelated to the selling off of school playing fields. Maternal lifestyle is also a very prominent contributor to the risk of obesity in the child, so targeting overweight and obese parents may be a better option. It has even been suggested that obesity in children should be made a child protection issue.

There has been a marked increase in the proportion of adults in the UK who are overweight or obese. In 1993 15 per cent were obese and 53 per cent either overweight or obese.[3] By 2019 these figures had risen to 28 per cent and 64 per cent. Globally, more than one billion adults are overweight, of whom some 300 million are obese.[4]

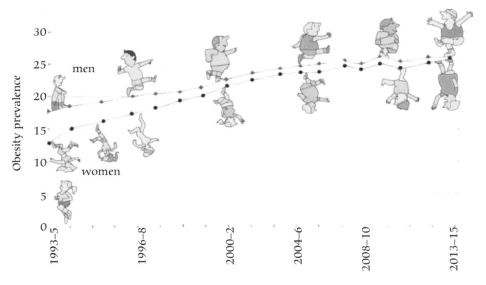

This huge increase in obesity would seem to be explained by the rise in availability of high-calorie foods, particularly sweet, fizzy drinks and the widespread use by the food industry of high-fructose corn syrup. Surprisingly, however, a team of economists from Holloway published a paper in 2016 showing that, judging by the sale of calorific foods, the average daily calorie intake of adults in the UK had actually fallen by 20 per cent over the previous 30 years![5] They concluded that the rise in obesity was a result of 'a decline in the strenuousness of work and daily life'. Their figures are supported by the Department for Food, Environment and Rural Affairs (DEFRA), which has shown that overall our calorie intake peaked in the 1970s, declined until the 2000s and has flattened since.[6] More evidence coming to similar conclusions is provided by the food surveys conducted by Public Health England. This view of the cause of our increasing obesity is not shared by all, however. The Obesity Health Alliance is firmly convinced that the causes are changes in diet, increased portion size, far more meals eaten outside the home and a shift to ready meals, junk food and snacks.[7] The whole problem is made more obtuse by the fact uncovered by the Office of National Statistics that the average Briton consumes 50 per cent more calories than they estimate for themselves – social-desirability bias again![8] As one representative of the National Obesity Forum is quoted as saying, 'People lie and I am not surprised that they do when it comes to food. They wish not to be taken for slobs, even though they may be just that!' As we have seen, the same bias results in a similar degree of overestimation of exercise taken – people take about 50–100 per cent less exercise than they claim. Moreover, the more overweight the individual, the greater the overestimate.[9]

Obesity is much more than a medical problem. In 2015 in the UK the cost to the NHS directly attributable to obesity was £4.2 billion and the cost to the wider economy was £27 billion. And as we get fatter our perceptions change: the new norm is to be overweight or obese, with the likely knock-on consequence of an increasingly corpulent population.

The medical ill effects of obesity

Obesity is not a disease, but it is a powerful risk factor for a number of dangerous illnesses, including such age-related conditions as lower-limb osteoarthritis, type 2 diabetes, dementia, hypertension, heart attacks, atrial fibrillation, strokes, oesophageal reflux, fatty liver and several varieties of cancer (uterus, breast, bowel, gullet, ovary, liver and pancreas for a start). The risk of dying from Covid-19 is doubled for obese patients.[10] Both quality of life and productivity are considerably reduced for the obese. Obesity also contributes significantly to disability in later life, making old people less able to carry out normal activities of daily living and more likely to become frail and dependent.[11] There is a reduction of about a quarter in disease-free life (healthspan – see page 155) in old age. Mortality rate increases by 30 per cent for every increment of 5 above a BMI of 25.[12] Yet, while 45 per cent of deaths of those with a BMI of 30 or more are due to obesity-related diseases, obesity is seldom recorded as a contributory factor on death certificates.[13]

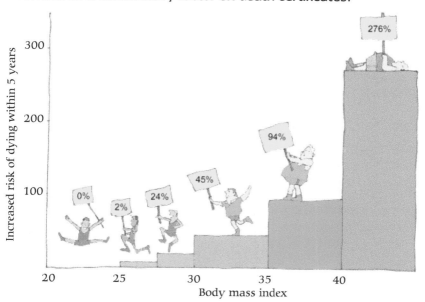

Increased risk of death over next five years with increasing BMI

A recent study of more than 10.5 million people over four continents has clarified the mortality risk of being overweight or obese. Compared with those of normal weight (BMI 20–25), having a BMI between 25 and 27.5 increases risk of death over the following five years by 7 per cent; a BMI between 27.5 and 30 increases risk by 20 per cent; a BMI between 30 and 35 increases risk by 45 per cent; a BMI between 35 and 40 increases risk by 94 per cent; and a BMI over 40 increases risk by a staggering 276 per cent.[14] It has been estimated that our obesity epidemic shortens lives by as many as nine years.

The risks are much greater for men than for women at all levels of obesity. About 1 in 7 premature deaths in Europe is due to being overweight or obese; overweight people lose on average one year of life; and obese people lose about three years of life. However, being thin is not always healthy. BMIs below 22 are also associated with increased mortality. It is presumed that thin people include those who are thin because they suffer ill health or practise unhealthy behaviour such as smoking.[15]

Other important ill effects of obesity include aggravation of breathlessness; worsening of asthma; damage to joints, particularly knees and hips; abnormal blood lipids; depression; and sleep apnoea. Wouldn't you do anything to avoid that lot? Either the answer is yes or you are not paying attention.

Exercise in the prevention of obesity

Staying a normal weight is much easier than losing weight. Those who take regular exercise from childhood seldom become obese.

Your weight is like your bank balance. Calories replace money, but with an opposite desirable outcome! Think of calories as cash – the more you put in as food, the richer or fatter you grow, while the more you take out as exercise, the poorer or thinner you become. Obesity is caused neither by a slow metabolism nor by big bones; it is caused by your energy intake being greater than your output. Some figures have been produced to illustrate the effectiveness of exercise in burning off excess calories. It has even been suggested that food packaging should include the exercise required to work off the contents! The labels would not make comfortable reading. Walking at between 3.5 and 4mph burns off about 5 calories per minute, so about 26 minutes of walking is needed to walk off a can of fizzy drink. A digestive biscuit might be used up by climbing 25 floors of stairs and a quarter of a pizza fuels running for 43 minutes.

Reaching a steady state with equal intake and output of calories is relatively easy if you are a regular exerciser. Hence the advantage of a good start – exercising from childhood.

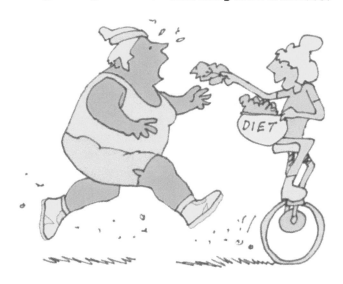

We do not know just how much exercise is needed to prevent obesity, nor to prevent weight being regained by those who have slimmed down. The figure of 60–90 minutes a day of moderately intense exercise has been calculated,[16] which is considerably more than the level recommended by the DoH for maintenance of good health. For runners, 15 miles per week seems to be the required load.[17] However, just as important as formal exercise for increasing energy output is the level of activity in day-to-day living. There is a host of ways in which you can increase your energy expenditure, including walking upstairs instead of taking the lift, walking up escalators, opting for active transport such as walking or cycling for getting to and from work, getting off the bus a stop earlier than your destination, walking short journeys rather than taking the car, etc., etc. Another important element in daily energy expenditure is the amount you fidget. People who fidget are thinner than those who don't and the energy expenditure of fidgeting can be as much as 600 Calories per day. Being a fidget has a strong inherited component and it may be difficult to make yourself into a fidgeter – though special fidget chairs have shown some promise.

Exercise in the treatment of obesity

Most adults in the developed world weigh too much and for them (you?) the problem is a difficult one. Getting rid of unwanted weight is much harder than avoiding putting it on in the first place. As anyone who has ever felt the need to go on a diet can tell you, it is *extremely* difficult to lose weight. Eating fewer calories than you expend in exercise is really, really hard – but it *can* be done. Some people have the willpower to cut their food intake to the level where they lose weight, but by the time we reach adulthood our dietary habits are hard-wired into us and most people who lose weight by diet alone subsequently put it all back on again.

Some people can increase their exercise level to the point where they lose weight, but this does need a lot of effort – you need to perform moderate-intensity exercise for an hour a day or run more than 15 miles per week to guarantee weight loss without changing what you eat. This makes sense when you realise that normal exercise regimes, which may take 150 minutes a week, are occupying only 2 per cent of your total waking hours. Increasing effort during these sessions makes a tiny contribution to your overall energy expenditure. Unfortunately, finding out how difficult it is to exercise your way out of obesity is demoralising and often results in giving up. You need to be realistic from the outset about how much exercise is needed.

The most successful weight-losing strategy is a combination of diet, exercise and, most important of all, maintenance of this changed lifestyle in perpetuity. Most people find it too difficult, perhaps because it means both taking an unaccustomed amount of exercise (which may increase the appetite) and being hungry. In a world where we are surrounded by too much high-calorie food, such self-denial may seem close to masochism.

The Cochrane Review on 'Exercise for Overweight or Obesity, 2006'[18] analysed the results of 43 studies involving 3,476 participants. Overall, they found exercise programmes without dietary changes produced a modest effect, with weight losses between 2kg and 7kg. More vigorous exercise was more effective than less vigorous. However, the most effective treatment was a combination of diet and exercise, with diet alone being rather more effective than exercise alone. A 24-year follow-up study of 116,564 women aged 30–55 found that the death rate in the inactive obese was two and a half times greater than in the lean active group.[19]

Those who exercise to lose weight achieve another benefit – a reduction in risk factors for cardiovascular disease, with lowering of blood pressure and blood sugar and an improvement in blood lipids. Improvements are seen even in those who take up exercise but fail to lose weight, a fact confirmed by studies showing that, while both BMI and fitness are strong independent predictors of all-cause mortality, fit obese patients have a lower mortality than unfit people of normal weight.[20] Alas, very few obese people take enough exercise to counteract the ill effects of obesity – one estimate calculated just 2.2 per cent of all men and 4.1 per cent of all women in England could be classed as both obese and fit.[21]

The other great benefit of using exercise as part of your weight-control programme is that it helps to maintain and increase your musculature – starvation diets are no respecters of which part of your body shrinks. Fat is not the only part to be diminished, as can be seen in the pictures of the victims of famines or wartime privation. Exercise training increases muscle mass – and muscle is somewhat more dense than fat. Those who fail to lose weight during exercise programmes may have lost fat but replaced it with muscle. One meta-analysis involving 4,815 subjects found that in the absence of weight loss, exercise produces a 6.1 per cent decrease in 'visceral adiposity' (i.e. paunch size), while diet showed virtually no change (1.1 per cent).[22]

The way you exercise has an influence on its effectiveness. Moderate-intensity exercise (MOD) has been compared with high-intensity interval (HIIT) and sprint-interval (SIT) training.[23] HIIT consists of short intervals of extreme exertion punctuated by rest periods. SIT is a more extreme form of HIIT. The primary difference between HIIT and SIT is that HIIT, despite what the name may suggest, reaches hard, but not *maximal* intensities, whereas SIT does require maximal and even supramaximal intensities. Studies have shown that all three regimes were associated with similar reductions in body-fat percentages, but interval training provided greater reductions in total fat mass. Since the time spent in MOD averaged 38 minutes, HIIT averaged 28 minutes and SIT averaged 18 minutes, the time saving of interval regimes might appeal to busy individuals.

Once weight has been lost by whatever combination of diet and exercise, there is a depressing tendency for the weight lost to be regained – more than 70 per cent of people who succeed in losing weight will have returned to their usual weight within two years.[24] It takes about 275 minutes per week of moderate exercise to maintain weight loss – considerably more than the DoH recommendations for healthy living. However, exercise is more effective than diet in maintaining weight loss.[25] Those who are successful in maintaining a lowered body weight eat more than unsuccessful dieters but expend significantly more energy in daily activity.

So the easiest way to lose weight is to combine eating less with exercising more. To keep it off, continuing the exercise habit is crucial. The trick, then, is to maintain your new lifestyle. There are a few determined souls who, having acknowledged the need to shed the pounds, are able to do so by willpower. For others, some doctors may prescribe pills, which might help a bit but only in the short term. Weight-losing groups such as WW (Weight Watchers) and Slimming World can be helpful. The only guaranteed way to keep weight off, however, is surgery. This is now available under the NHS in a limited range of circumstances – but what a way to manage what is after all a lifestyle choice.

There has been a move in the medical profession to label obesity as 'an ongoing chronic disease' and to reduce the 'shaming' of fat people. Rather, we are encouraged to sympathise with fat people for the 'health inequalities, genetic influences and social factors' that have contributed to their problem. This philosophy is more common in the US than in the UK. However, I disagree with this approach – how can anyone who believes that they are a victim of uncontrollable outside forces come to understand that they can change their own situation for the better?

High Blood Pressure (Hypertension)

My doctors told me this morning my blood pressure is down so low that I can start reading the newspapers. Ronald Reagan

High blood pressure is another risk factor – mainly for coronary disease and stroke. Blood pressure (BP) is expressed as a two-figure quantity – say, 120/80. The higher figure is the systolic pressure, which is the peak pressure reached when blood is

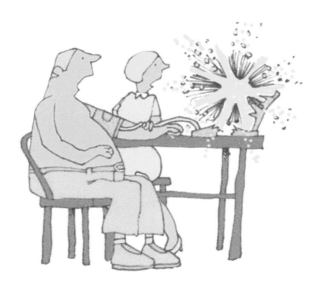

pumped out from the heart to the main arteries. The arterial pressure then falls to the lower figure, which is the diastolic pressure, the lowest level reached before it is pushed up again by the next contraction of the heart. A level of 140/90 or less is usually taken as normal. The unit of measurement used is millimetres of mercury, mmHg. This is a strangely antique unit which came into being because blood pressure was always measured with a mercury 'sphygmomanometer' (a BP-measuring instrument) that uses the height of a column of mercury as the measure of pressure. Modern sphygmomanometers no longer use mercury, so it would be more logical to use the Système International (SI) unit of pressure, the Pascal. However, the long-established mmHg is so ingrained into doctors' psyche that they have clung on to this archaic unit, rather as we continue to measure distance in the UK in miles rather than kilometres.

The distribution of blood pressure (BP) in the population follows the usual distribution of most human characteristics – the bell-shaped curve. As with height, for instance, there are a few people at the lower end of the range and a few at the upper end, but most are somewhere in between.

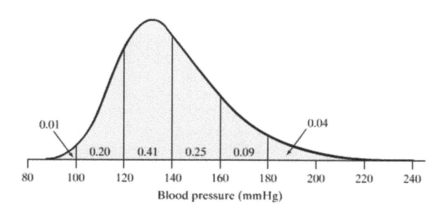

Range of systolic blood pressure in the population, taking the Gaussian or bell-shaped distribution

For the majority, high blood pressure is not a disease – just the top end of a continuous scale. For a few, high BP is due to some other condition, particularly kidney disease. Someone deemed by the medical profession to have high blood pressure is labelled as having 'hypertension'. It is a very difficult condition to define – just where is the cut-off between acceptable upper level of blood pressure and unacceptable hypertension? It could be the level above which the complications of raised blood pressure kick in – but unfortunately the ill effects develop insidiously and the higher your pressure the higher the risk. Wallis Simpson said that 'you can never be too thin or too rich' and to that I would add 'nor have too low a blood pressure'.

A better definition of hypertension would be the level above which lowering the blood pressure reduces risk. Here we should be on firmer ground, but unfortunately even this soil is somewhat boggy. For decades it has been assumed that when a mildly raised pressure is treated with the appropriate medication to reach a more pleasing figure, risk is automatically reduced. However, there has been no evidence for reducing the level below 140 systolic until a recent study from the US, the SPRINT study, which has indicated that getting the pressure down to 120 systolic may have substantial advantages over the higher target of 140.[1] There is less certainty about appropriate BP levels in people over the age of 80. Enthusiastic lowering of BP in this group carries the risk of postural hypotension – low BP when standing.[2] This may cause faintness, dizziness and possibly dangerous falls in the elderly. It may also aggravate cognitive decline in older people.[3]

Another confusion in the assessment of blood pressure is that it is not a fixed figure; it is a fiction of the moment. It varies with time of day, pressure of work, timing of meals and contact with other people – particularly doctors. We are all aware of 'white coat' hypertension, which is the condition in which blood pressure is markedly higher when measured by a doctor. If you want to know what your blood pressure really is, take it yourself. There are plenty of reliable automatic home blood-pressure machines which will give you a much more accurate picture of your BP, at whatever time of day you wish, than does the occasional snapshot BP taken in the surgery. The alternative is the 24-hour blood pressure recorder which is available in most GP surgeries.

However it is measured, raised blood pressure is common in Western societies and it continues to rise steadily with age. A recent American study found the prevalence of hypertension to be 9 per cent for those aged 18–44, 40 per cent for those aged 45–64 and 75 per cent for those aged 65 and over.[4]

The medical ill effects of raised BP

Persistently raised blood pressure damages the walls of the arteries and this predisposes the person to atheroma, or hardening of the arteries (see page 100). This is a narrowing of the blood vessels by patchy plaques, which build up over many years, reducing the internal dimensions – or lumen – of the vessels and sometimes leading to complete blockage. The most damaging results include heart attacks, strokes and, less commonly, gangrene of the legs. Other ill effects of hypertension include kidney failure, heart failure and vascular dementia. Hypertension is the largest of all the risk factors for stroke, responsible for about 54 per cent of cases. It is also an important risk factor for heart attacks, being implicated in about 47 per cent of cases.[5]

Exercise in the prevention of raised blood pressure

Physical fitness has a direct effect on blood pressure. A large Harvard alumni study showed that those who engaged in regular vigorous leisure activities had a 33 per cent lower risk of developing hypertension than those who took little exercise.[6] There is a dose-response relationship between physical fitness and BP – that is to say, the fitter you are, the lower your BP is likely to be. In a study of 5,249 middle-aged males in Copenhagen, every increase in VO_{2max} of 10ml/min/kg was associated with a 2mmHg reduction in both systolic and diastolic BP.[7] A study that examined exactly which form of sport or exercise was most effective found that running, tennis, team sports, exercise classes and resistance training were best for keeping BP low.[8] More specifically, regular muscle-strengthening lowers the risk of developing hypertension by about 60 per cent.[9]

Exercise in the treatment of raised blood pressure

Whatever your BP may be, you would probably be better off if, by your own efforts, you could bring it down. There are many aspects of lifestyle that contribute to pushing up your BP. The most important are eating too much salt, drinking too much alcohol, being obese and, surprise, surprise, taking too little exercise. So you would probably benefit from cutting down salt and alcohol, losing weight and increasing your exercise level. Exercise as simple as walking reduces BP and the higher your BP, the greater the effect. A single bout of exercise reduces BP for several hours, while exercise training reduces BP both at rest and during exercise.[10] This training effect is reflected in a dose-related lowering of the risk of cardiovascular disease and premature death at all degrees of hypertension – in other words, the more exercise that is taken, the lower the rate of both CVD and premature death.[11]

After an extensive appraisal of the evidence, the American College of Cardiology concluded that for adult men and women regular aerobic physical activity decreases systolic and diastolic pressure significantly: 'The amount of physical activity recommended for lowering BP is congruent with the amount of physical activity recommended in 2008 by the federal government for overall health. Most health benefits occur with at least 150 minutes a week of moderate intensity physical activity such as brisk walking. *Additional benefits occur with more physical activity*' [my emphasis].[12]

No trial has directly compared the effect of exercise with that of medication in reducing BP. However, comparative analysis of many trials of both approaches has indicated that exercise does have a very similar effect on blood pressure as medication.[13] The largest meta-analysis carried out compared the results of medication in 29,000 subjects with exercise in 10,000 subjects and concluded that at an individual patient basis medication was slightly more effective, but in groups the average showed no difference.[14]

The effect of exercise on blood pressure is greatest in those who already have hypertension. It is likely that reducing your BP with exercise and other lifestyle changes, such as losing weight and cutting back on salt and alcohol, are more effective at reducing risk than taking pills. Each lifestyle change has many other benefits. Often these can reduce BP sufficiently to allow the previously hypertensive patient to stop taking medication. The American Heart Association has summarised the benefits of exercise as well as other treatments in the management of high blood pressure,[15] concluding that 'moderate-intensity dynamic aerobic regimens are capable of significantly lowering BP among most individuals within a few months.' It also appears that hypertension that is resistant to medication can respond to exercise training.[16]

Dyslipidaemia

It is a scientific fact that your body will not absorb cholesterol
if you take it from someone else's plate.
Dave Barry, writer and humorist

Please forgive me for giving you such a dreadful word – it means undesirable changes in your blood fats. This is a complicated field and I am going to greatly oversimplify it. Please don't quote any of this back to a lipid specialist, or, if you do, say you found it in *Reader's Digest*.

There are a number of different forms of fat in the bloodstream and the form you will have heard most about is cholesterol. Cholesterol is an important component of cell walls – we all need it if we are to function properly. The cholesterol in the blood is carried by proteins called lipoproteins and can be very roughly divided into two forms – low-density lipoprotein cholesterol (LDL-C) and high-density lipoprotein cholesterol (HDL-C). LDL-C is available for laying down in the walls of the arteries in the plaques of atheroma, or hardening of the arteries – the pinch-points that narrow the artery. This is 'bad' cholesterol. HDL-C is being carried to the liver, where it is broken down and excreted in the bile. This is 'good' cholesterol. A high level of LDL-C is a risk factor for atheroma, leading to heart attacks and strokes.

There are various causes of high LDL-C, including genetic factors, being overweight, having an underactive thyroid gland, some forms of kidney disease and eating a high-fat diet, particularly a diet with a lot of 'saturated' fat. Saturated fat is largely derived from animals – cream, butter, fatty joints of meat and, particularly, prepared meat products such as meat pies, patés and sausages. Fat is cheaper than lean meat, so food manufacturers use it liberally.

A high level of HDL-C protects against atheroma. The main cause of low HDL-C is physical inactivity and the most effective way of increasing this fat fraction is by regular vigorous exercise.

The 'normal' levels of these fat fractions is somewhat arbitrary and there is a tendency for each new generation of cholesterol police to set the limits for total cholesterol and LDL-C lower and lower. Currently the recommended upper limit for total cholesterol is 5.0mmol/litre and for LDL-C it is 3.0. The bell-shaped curve of normal distribution would put most of the population in the too-high category. HDL-C makes up around one quarter of the total cholesterol – the current recommendation is that it should be above 1.0mmol/l. A better measure of risk for atheroma and cardiovascular disease is the ratio between HDL-C and total cholesterol. This should be below 4.0 and preferably much lower. This is the measure of cholesterol level used in algorithms for calculating risk of CVD ('Q-Risk3'; see www.qrisk.org).

The treatment of dyslipidaemia should involve changes in diet, but in practice most people find it nearly impossible to change the way they eat and maintain it. The modern treatment is the group of drugs known as the statins – and very effective they are too. Not only do they reduce LDL-C by up to 30 per cent and also reduce the LDL/HDL ratio, but they reduce the risk of atheroma substantially – so substantially that it is regarded as obligatory to prescribe them to all those deemed to be at high risk and particularly to those who already have evidence of arterial disease.

The medical ill effects of dyslipidaemia

This is all about disease of the arterial system – atheroma, or hardening of the arteries. Both a high total cholesterol and a high ratio of total cholesterol to HDL cholesterol are powerful risk factors for heart attacks, strokes and peripheral vascular disease (see page 119). For this reason the total cholesterol/HDL-C ratio is an important element of the Q-Risk assessment for predicting CVD. Dyslipidaemia is also a feature of the 'metabolic syndrome' (see page 108), which is a combination of obesity, hypertension, diabetes and lipid abnormalities. The metabolic syndrome carries a high risk of CVD, particularly heart disease.

Effect of exercise on lipids

Here I fear I am leading you into choppy seas – the answer to just what effect exercise has on the different fat fractions found in the blood is very unclear.

There are age-related changes in total cholesterol and LDL cholesterol, both of which increase gradually with time. A study of physical fitness in 11,400 people who had several treadmill tests over 36 years found those in the lower third for fitness developed abnormal lipids 10–15 years earlier than those in the fittest third.[1] In other words, it does seem that regular exercise delays the age-related development of undesirable changes in blood fats. This idea is supported by the finding that regular walking reduces both the total cholesterol and the all-important ratio of total cholesterol to HDL-C.[2]

The data on the response of lipid abnormalities to exercise alone are surprisingly and disappointingly sparse, and sometimes contradictory. A 2005 meta-analysis concluded that regular aerobic exercise does raise HDL-C levels,[3] but that the effect on other lipid levels was less certain. It also seemed that exercise alone was less effective than the combination of diet and exercise.[4] However, a more recent meta-analysis from 2011 confusingly found that diet and exercise reduces total cholesterol, total cholesterol/HDL-C ratio and LDL-C but has little effect on the protective HDL-C.[5] So, a bit of disparity there, but all are agreed that regular exercise does reduce the all-important total cholesterol/HDL-C ratio.

Perhaps the most effective management of dyslipidaemia is the combination of statins with exercise. In a cohort of 10,043 Americans with dyslipidaemia, among men treated with statins the risk of dying over the next 10 years for the most fit was just 30 per cent of the risk for the least fit.[6]

Finally, take heed of the conclusions of the American Heart Association and the American College of Cardiology. After a thorough appraisal of all the evidence, they concluded that it may require 12 MET task hours per week of exercise to lower LDL-C.[7] How much is that? About 1 hour 40 minutes per week of very brisk walking (4mph). Get to it!

Diabetes

There are really only two requirements when it comes to exercise. One is that you do it. The other is that you continue to do it.
from The New Glucose Revolution for Diabetes

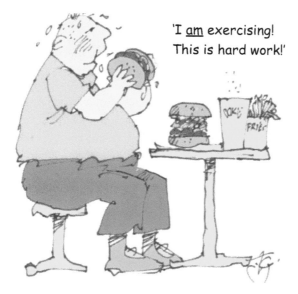

'I am exercising! This is hard work!'

Type 2 diabetes mellitus (T2DM) is what we are talking about. Type 1 DM is something else, although it is also a risk factor for cardiovascular disease. T1DM is a condition whose onset is usually in young people whose pancreas fairly suddenly packs in and stops producing insulin.

Insulin is essential for the control of sugar in the blood, ushering the sugar into the cells to help fuel activity and ensuring that the level of glucose in the blood is kept within narrow limits. Type 1 diabetics can survive only by regularly injecting themselves with insulin for the rest of their days. T2DM develops later in life and is largely a result of an unhealthy lifestyle. There is a genetic element – the tendency to develop T2DM is inherited, but it rarely manifests in the absence of too much food and too little exercise. The pancreas in normal people responds to the flood of glucose into the bloodstream after each meal by increasing the output of insulin. The insulin helps the cells to absorb the glucose, keeping blood glucose level constant and fuelling cellular activity. Exercise assists this process by enhancing absorption of glucose into muscle cells.

People who carry too much weight, particularly those with central obesity, and take too little exercise develop a state called insulin resistance. In this condition, insulin becomes less effective at keeping blood glucose levels normal and a greater production of insulin is needed to maintain homeostasis (normal blood levels). So the pancreas has to work ever harder to produce enough insulin for normal metabolism and eventually becomes unable to satisfy the body's ability to keep its sugar level within normal limits – blood sugar rises, known as 'hyperglycaemia', the hallmark of diabetes, in this case T2DM. The problem is aggravated by the laying down of fat where it is not wanted. In the liver this further increases insulin resistance. In the pancreas it further reduces the production of insulin.

Diabetes is a growing epidemic, with ever-rising rates of diagnosis as the population becomes older and fatter – and lazier. Obesity accounts for about 80 per cent of the risk of developing T2DM. In the mid-1990s about 2–3 per cent of the UK population were known to be affected; the figure now is about 6 per cent and growing,[1] with about 100,000 newly diagnosed diabetics each year. There are about 4 million diabetic patients in the UK, with more than 21,000 deaths per annum. With the enormous increase in childhood obesity, T2DM in children, which used to be a rarity, is on the rise too. In England and Wales about 7,000 people under the age of 25 are diabetic (Diabetes UK figures). The cost to the NHS of managing diabetes is a staggering £11.7 billion,[2] which is more than 12 per cent of the total NHS budget.

Side effects of diabetes

The complications of diabetes are legion. It is a risk factor for atheroma ('hardening of the arteries') of large vessels, which leads to heart attacks and strokes and may result in gangrene of the legs. Small blood vessels are also affected, leading to impairment of sight and ultimately to blindness. Damage to nerves causes numbness and neuralgic pain. Other ill effects include kidney disease and susceptibility to infections. Since most type 2 diabetics are obese, they are at increased risk of a number of different cancers, but there is also a link between diabetes and cancer that is independent of their obesity. Untreated diabetes is also a risk factor for dementia, which develops more rapidly in diabetic sufferers, and frailty is an increasing end-stage for many.

T2DM is not a nice disease and in most cases it is preventable. Indeed, too much food and too little exercise are such important causative factors that diabetes can be cured in a proportion of sufferers simply by doing more and eating less.[3] The fact that this is so seldom achieved is a tribute to the difficulty in getting inactive, overweight individuals to change their lifestyles. Part of the problem may lie in the fact that so many diabetics seem to be unaware that they have the cure for their disease in their own hands.

Exercise in the prevention of diabetes

A number of studies have confirmed that diet and exercise reduce the chance of developing T2DM in susceptible people (i.e. obese people or those with insulin resistance) to less than half the expected level.[4-6] For them, a weight loss of 13 per cent reduces the risk of progressing to diabetes by 40 per cent. Diabetic risk is reduced in proportion to the amount of exercise taken – up to a level of 22 MET hours per week.[7] When it comes to specific exercise types, running, cycling, resistance training and yoga have all been found to be effective.[8] Exercise is also as effective as medication for preventing the progression from 'pre-diabetes' to clinical T2DM.[9]

It is difficult to disentangle the effects of diet and exercise in this condition which is so dependent on body weight. We can, however, be sure that any intervention that reduces body weight – which certainly includes exercise (see above) – will also reduce the incidence of T2DM. Some studies of exercise as preventative treatment have shown that almost any level of activity is beneficial, though with smaller gains for increased effort at higher levels of exertion.[10] Curiously, leisure-time activity is more effective than occupational exertion.[11]

The latest Cochrane Review looked at 12 randomised controlled trials (RCTs) of diet and exercise for over 5,000 people at high risk of T2DM.[12] The review concluded that the effects of diet or exercise alone were relatively small, but the combination did have a significant effect, reducing the risk from 26 per cent in the control group to 15 per cent in the combined group. Additional benefits of this approach to prevention are reduction in weight, waist circumference and blood pressure.

Exercise in the treatment of diabetes

As for prevention, diet and exercise should be the centrepieces of any treatment for diabetes – aiming to reduce weight and thereby lessen insulin resistance. If this is done quickly and effectively, many patients with diabetes are cured.[13] Studies of diet and exercise in the treatment of T2DM have indicated that up to nearly 50 per cent can be cured of their disease in this way.[14] The most successful RCT of lifestyle management of T2DM was reported from Scotland and Newcastle in 2018, with 298 obese diabetic patients receiving either intensive weight management or their usual care. The intervention group had their medication withdrawn, were given a carefully controlled diet, completely different from the one they usually ate, for a period of 12 weeks, followed by a 4-week food-reintroduction phase and a further weight-management phase lasting up to 2 years, using diet and exercise programmes to try to prevent them regaining weight. After one year, 46 per cent of the intervention group had remission of their diabetes compared with only 4 per cent in the control group.[15] There was a reduction of an amazing 86 per cent in the incidence of diabetes among those who lost 15kg or more.

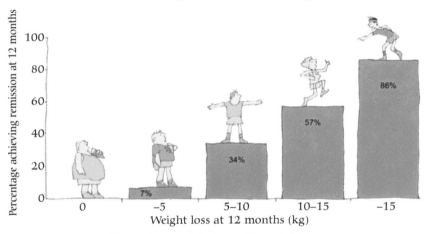

Remission of diabetes with weight loss

For some, such an approach is too late to effect a cure – the pancreas is already exhausted and cannot keep up with the body's demands. Nevertheless, diet and exercise enhance the effects of other treatments and sometimes make them unnecessary. Most diabetics need tablets to reduce their blood sugar to reasonable levels and some require insulin. Diet and exercise, combined with weekly counselling, have been shown to reduce considerably the need for medication even in those not cured.[16] Results were best for those who lost the most weight or who started the programme with less severe or with newly diagnosed diabetes. Regular exercise improves blood-sugar control, improves blood lipids, lowers blood pressure and increases physical fitness.[17] Better sexual function and quality of life are additional benefits.[18]

Exercise in the prevention of the complications of diabetes

Intensive lifestyle interventions have many other benefits for the type 2 diabetic. These include better glucose and lipid control, improved blood pressure, less sleep apnoea, lower liver fat, less depression, less urinary incontinence, less severe kidney disease and less retinopathy (i.e. blindness and sight loss), reduced need of diabetes medications, maintenance of physical mobility, improved quality of life, less knee pain, improved sexual function, lowered inflammation and reduced overall health costs.[19] Exercise also increases life expectancy for diabetics.[20]

What a tragedy: the world is full of overweight and obese diabetics treating their overeating and under-exercising with pills and sometimes injections. I wonder how many diabetics, facing a lifetime (a shortened lifetime at that) of treatment and unnecessary complications, realise that regular exercise and appropriate diet can both prevent and cure their disease.

The Metabolic Syndrome

Your genetics load the gun. Your lifestyle pulls the trigger.
Mehmet Oz

'What's that?' I hear you cry. Well, it is a rather important cluster of some of the conditions that have been described above and which make you particularly prone to arterial problems, particularly coronary disease. There are five components of the metabolic syndrome, also known as 'Syndrome X' – abdominal or central obesity, raised blood pressure, insulin resistance (pre-diabetes), raised blood triglycerides (a fat fraction) and low HDL cholesterol (see Dyslipidaemia, page 100). If you've got three or more of these you have the metabolic syndrome,[1] with insulin resistance appearing to be its major component.

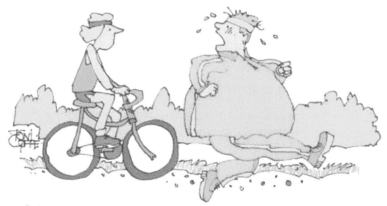

'I'm trying to outrun the metabolic syndrome . . . well, as far as the pub!'

The metabolic syndrome (MetSyn) has been recognised for the past 50 years or so. It is caused by a combination of unhealthy (over-)eating, lack of exercise, sedentary behaviour, getting older and being under stress. It is common, affecting about one in four adults in the UK. Approximately 50 per cent of heart-attack patients have the syndrome and it increases the risk of dying from heart disease about threefold.[2]

Exercise in the prevention of the metabolic syndrome

Since lack of exercise is an important risk factor for developing the MetSyn, it does not require a genius to work out that taking exercise is a sensible way of keeping the condition at bay – and so it has been demonstrated. In the Ely Study of 604 healthy middle-aged men and women followed up for 5.6 years, objectively measured physical activity predicted the development of MetSyn in a dose-dependent way – i.e. the less exercise taken, the higher the risk of the syndrome.[3] The beneficial effect of exercise in this respect is found at all levels of obesity.[4]

Similarly, the level of physical fitness, which itself is largely determined by levels of physical activity, is a strong predictor of MetSyn. In a study of fitness levels in 9,666 men aged 20–69, the overall prevalence of the syndrome was 25 per cent and the unfit men were twice as likely to have MetSyn as the fit men.[5] When the association has been studied in older men and women it has been found to be even more dramatic. MetSyn is up to 10 times more common in the unfit compared with the very fit.[6]

Exercise in the treatment of the metabolic syndrome

Exercise is effective in improving each one of the components of the metabolic syndrome – so again, no surprises to hear that exercise has been shown to be effective in treating the whole syndrome. One trial of exercise in 621 apparently healthy but sedentary individuals found that 105 had MetSyn at the start of the programme and 32 of these were free of the syndrome by its end. Improvements in all components were found.[7] There is evidence of an exercise-dose relationship, with high-dose, vigorous-intensity exercise, such as hard running, cycling or swimming, being more effective than lower doses.[8]

Coronary Heart Disease (CHD)

Except for the occasional heart attack I never felt better.
Dick Cheney, former US vice-president

The coronary arteries are the vessels that take blood to the heart muscle. They arise from the root of the aorta, the body's main artery, and wind round the surface of the heart in the shape of an upside-down papal crown or corona – hence their name. Their function is to supply the heart muscle with oxygen and nutrition.

Coronary artery disease is the narrowing of one or more of the coronary arteries, thus reducing the rate at which blood can flow through the artery. Coronary artery disease, more usually referred to as coronary heart disease (CHD), was until very recently the commonest cause of death in most developed societies (now narrowly overtaken in the UK by dementia for women). In the UK approximately 2.3 million people have diagnosed CHD, with around 300,000 new cases every year. About 200 people in the UK die of CHD every day, mainly from heart attacks.[1] It is also a cause of much morbidity – the symptoms and limitations resulting from the disease.

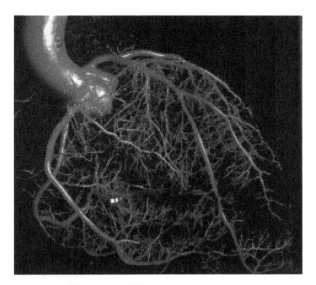

Wax cast of the coronary arteries

Coronary artery disease does not have a single cause: a number of 'risk factors' contribute to its development. Some are irreversible – age (the older you are, the more susceptible you are); gender (men develop CHD on average 10 years younger than women); and family history (you are at greater risk if you have a close relative with the disease, and the younger that relative, the greater the risk to you). You can't do anything about these risk factors, but you *can* tackle the reversible factors – cigarette-smoking, high blood pressure, diabetes, high blood cholesterol and obesity (and their combination: see The Metabolic Syndrome, page 108). Overshadowing all of these, because it contributes to most of them, is lack of exercise.

There are several tools for predicting the risk of developing CHD in any individual. The best validated is the Q-Risk 3. Go online at https://qrisk.org/three/. You will be asked to feed in your age, sex, height, weight, cholesterol/HDL ratio, blood pressure, presence or not of diabetes, ethnicity, smoking status, family history, deprivation, BMI, presence of rheumatoid arthritis or kidney disease, and postcode. Don't worry if you do not know all of these. The risk-scoring system will just give you average values for missing data. From that information, the tool will calculate your risk of developing both CHD and cardiovascular disease (CVD) over the next 10 years.

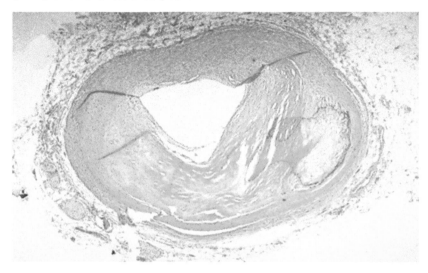

Diseased coronary artery under the microscope

Angina

Arterial narrowing is caused by a process called atheroma, or 'hardening of the arteries' (see also Dyslipidaemia, page 100). As we grow older we develop patchy narrowing of the arteries due to fatty plaques composed of cholesterol being laid down in the arterial wall and compounded by overlying thin layers of blood clot. This gradually restricts the flow of blood to the heart muscle. A point may be reached when the artery is unable to supply the needs of the heart muscle during exercise – the muscle lacks a sufficient supply of oxygen to be able to continue to contract effectively and this produces pain during exertion – *angina pectoris*. This is a tight, strangling pain across the centre of the chest, often radiating into the throat, jaws or left arm. It forces the sufferer to stop exercising and then settles over the next few minutes.

Heart attack

The atheroma plaques are delicate creatures and may break, crack or burst. If this happens, the body's repair mechanisms are set off and that usually means that a clot forms. This is a *coronary thrombosis* and may be large enough to block the artery. The result is death of the area of heart muscle supplied by that artery – *myocardial infarction*. This is what we usually call a heart attack. The immediate danger is sudden death due to rhythm disturbance precipitated by the damage to the heart muscle. For those who survive to reach hospital, the outlook is good.

Heart failure

The modern treatment of heart attacks is extremely effective in limiting the damage done. Even so, if there is enough loss of myocardium (heart muscle), particularly after more than one attack, the ability of the heart to perform its full function is damaged. This can lead to heart failure. The term 'heart failure' sounds dire, but does not mean the end of life. It simply means that the heart is too weak to deliver all its potential output in daily activities. This causes fatigue, poor circulation with cold hands and feet, breathlessness on exertion and inability to carry out the tasks of daily living. If inadequately treated, it may cause ankle-swelling and breathlessness while at rest or when lying down at night.

Exercise in the prevention of CHD

Back in the 1950s and 1960s, studies of bus drivers[2] and Whitehall civil servants[3] by Jerry Morris, a Scottish doctor working at University College, London, became epidemiological classics. In the former, he and his colleagues compared the rates of heart disease in London bus drivers with those of bus conductors. While the drivers sat all day long, fuming at pesky taxi drivers and other road-users, the conductors shinned up and down stairs getting plenty of exercise. They found that the drivers had a more than 40 per cent higher rate of CHD than the conductors.

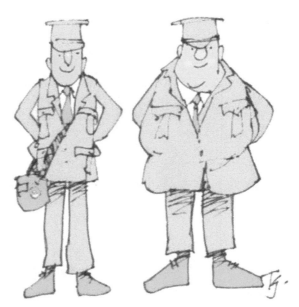

Guess who's the bus driver?

The Whitehall civil servant study looked at leisure-time physical activity and again found that the rate of fatal heart attacks in those who took vigorous exercise as recreation was about 40 per cent that of the inactive, while the rate of non-fatal heart attacks was 50 per cent. Morris made several discoveries: that intermittent heavy exercise is more effective than lower-level activity, even with equivalent totals of exercise; that there is a threshold for the protective effect; and there is dose-response relationship above this level – i.e. the more exercise you take, the better the effect. I will discuss the application of these trial data to mortality in Chapter 12.

In the USA, similar studies were carried out on the San Francisco longshore men (stevedores) and on university graduates.[4, 5] In a study of nearly 17,000 Harvard graduates aged 35–74, they found that taking exercise was inversely related to mortality – that is to say, the more exercise taken the greater the reduction in mortality. A further study from the US followed over 26,000 men and women who had performed an exercise test to determine their levels of physical fitness.[6] They divided the subjects by fitness level – high, moderate and low. Over an average follow-up of 10 years, the rate of coronary disease was 11 per cent lower in the moderate-fitness group and 25 per cent lower in the high-fitness group when compared to the low-fitness group.

Since then numerous studies have confirmed the association between regular exercise, physical fitness and protection from CHD.[7] They have shown that the greater the total of physical activity, running, weight training and rowing, the greater the reduction in the risk of CHD.[8] Also, improving fitness level from unfit to fit nearly halves risk compared with remaining unfit.[9] Most tellingly, a meta-analysis of 33 trials, which included over 100,000 subjects followed up for an average of 11 years after an exercise test (see Chapter 12), divided them into low-, intermediate- and high-fitness categories. The low-fitness group had a 56 per cent higher chance of suffering a heart attack than the high-fitness group.[10]

The beneficial effects of exercise holds for all age groups that have been investigated.[11,12] It has been estimated that if everyone were physically active, 6 per cent of coronary disease worldwide would be eliminated and life expectancy of the world population would be increased by 0.68 years.[13]

Even the rather limited doses of exercise recommended by national bodies (see page 63) are protective. In a study of nearly half a million adults in the USA, compliance with exercise guidelines was compared with mortality over nine years. For those following the recommendations for strength-building, the death rate was 82 per cent of that expected; for those following the aerobic exercise recommendations it was 65 per cent; and for those following both it was 50 per cent.[14]

Some of the ways in which exercise prevents CHD are obvious. Most of the reversible risk factors are reduced. Regular exercisers are thinner than non-exercisers, have lower blood pressure, lower blood cholesterol and are less likely to develop diabetes. Apart from stopping smoking, if you do, there is no more effective way of avoiding a heart attack than regular vigorous exercise.

Exercise in the treatment of CHD

The use of exercise for treating CHD preceded its use for treating any other non-communicable disease, often abbreviated to NCD. Back in the 18th century Dr William Heberden recognised angina and in 1768 he described one of his patients, who had been cured by sawing wood for half an hour a day.[15]

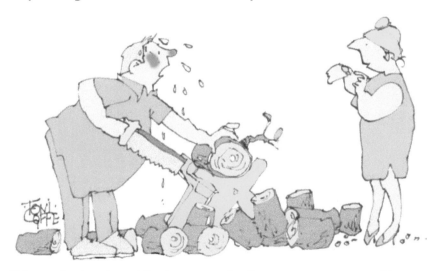

'I know what's going on! Is this a way of telling me you want central heating?'

CHD, however, was infrequently diagnosed over the next 150 years and by the time it became accepted as a serious health problem, early in the 20th century, this lesson had been forgotten. When a heart attack was diagnosed, prolonged bed rest was thought to be essential if the patient's life were to be saved – it was believed that exertion too soon after the attack risked rupturing the damaged heart. Doctors and nurses went to absurd lengths to keep the patient at complete 'rest' for several weeks, spoon-feeding them and insisting on the use of that most exercise-intensive utensil, the bedpan! When the patient was eventually released from hospital, the advice was for exercise to be restricted in favour of a peaceful, sedentary life.

In the 1940s and 1950s some of the undesirable consequences of bed-rest were being appreciated – deconditioning, boredom, depression, venous thrombosis and chest infection to mention just a few. The idea of early mobilisation was gaining credibility. In Cleveland, Ohio, a farseeing cardiologist called Herman Hellerstein and his colleagues developed a comprehensive rehabilitation programme with graduated exercise training as its centrepiece. The idea was to 'add life to years and perhaps years to life' for 'habitually sedentary, lazy, hypokinetic, sloppy, endo-mesomorphic overweight males' through a programme of enhanced physical activity.[16] (Dr Hellerstein appears to have held his coronary patients in high regard!) They showed that patients who had recovered from a heart attack could have their physical fitness improved, ECG changes recorded during and after exertion reduced and psychological status raised by a course of exercise to which they added improvement in nutrition, giving up smoking and continuation of gainful employment and normal social life.[17]

Over the past 50 years there have been numerous controlled trials of cardiac rehabilitation in patients recovering from such events as heart attacks or heart surgery, and meta-analyses of the results have indicated a fall in the region of 25 per cent in the mortality rate in treated groups over the subsequent three years. Interestingly, when exercise-only programmes have been compared with more comprehensive programmes, the exercise-only treatments fare as well as those offering in addition counselling, education and risk-factor advice.[18,19] It is my belief that it is extremely difficult to change the behaviour of the middle-aged and the only advice that has much chance of making an impact is that concerning exercise – particularly when it is incorporated into patient management.

In patients with established CHD, exercise capacity remains a powerful predictor of prognosis. For every 1 MET reduction in fitness there is an increased risk of death of 13 per cent.[20] One study has shown that mortality in CHD patients with a VO_{2max} of less than 15 is more than double that of those with a VO_{2max} of more than 22 in those followed up for an average of 8 years.[21] Indeed, physical fitness in CHD patients is a better predictor of future mortality than any other measure. This effect is partly because low fitness reflects greater heart damage; even so, increasing fitness with exercise training reduces mortality risk to the level of untrained subjects with an equivalent fitness level.

Unfortunately, the application of this knowledge is not as good as it might be. The level of exercise and the length of the exercise component of cardiac rehabilitation in the UK is well below that of the programmes used to show their benefits. A recent study showed that, in a sample of 70 coronary patients receiving the usual twice-weekly exercise course for eight weeks, there was no increase in fitness level and no reduction in five-year mortality.[22] A further failure of our care of heart patients was shown by a study of 4,000 people recovering from a coronary event from the previous two years: 45 per cent were still smoking, 36 per cent were obese, 53 per cent had central obesity and 52 per cent were classified as inactive.[23]

Exercise in the treatment of heart failure

As discussed above, one important consequence of cardiac damage from coronary disease is heart failure. In this condition the ability of the heart to pump out enough blood for daily living is impaired, with resulting tiredness, breathlessness and restriction of activities. There are about 900,000 people living with heart failure in the UK.

The more the heart is damaged, the less effect any physical training has on its function. With heart failure it is still possible to increase physical fitness, but this is through peripheral training effects – improved muscular efficiency and blood-flow distribution. The exercise training of patients with heart failure is further restricted by the limited exercise intensity and dose that they can sustain. Exercise training of heart-failure patients can be helpful but must be increased slowly and carefully. The resulting benefits are modest.

A meta-analysis of RCTs of exercise training for 4,400 heart-failure patients found an increase in timed walking distance of about 6 per cent, which is enough to be beneficial.[24] Quality of life scores increased slightly and there was no increase in either hospital admission or mortality.

Peripheral Vascular Disease

Used to be rock around the clock, now it's limp about the block.
Anon.

Atheroma ('hardening') can involve any part of the vascular tree. Arterial disease of the legs is called peripheral vascular disease (PVD). The main risk factors are diabetes (see page 103), cigarette-smoking, high blood pressure (see page 95) and dyslipidaemia (see page 100). In a minority there is a strong inherited predisposition.

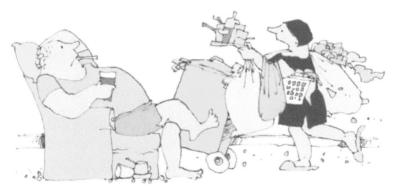

'You've got P.V.D.? More like L.A.Z.Y. if you ask me.'

PVD affects about 10 per cent of diabetics at 10 years after diagnosis, rising to 45 per cent at 20 years. The incidence in non-diabetics is between 5 and 10 per cent for over-65-year-olds. Like coronary disease, PVD initially causes muscle pain on exertion –

usually pain in the calf when walking, resolving rapidly on stopping. Just like angina, but in the leg muscles instead of the heart muscle. This is called intermittent *claudication*, or intermittent limping, named after the emperor Claudius, a famous limper. Progression of the arterial narrowing may lead to blockage and severe lack of blood to the feet. The lower parts of the legs may develop ulcers which won't heal. Toes become painful, then white and ultimately black and gangrenous, requiring amputation. If you are diabetic, please don't smoke.

Penile blood supply may also be affected by PVD, causing erectile dysfunction. Erections are absent, weak or cannot be sustained – a cause of much distress and frustration to those so afflicted.

Exercise in the prevention of PVD

Regular exercise improves arterial elasticity and lessens arterial stiffness. This was shown in a study of middle-aged first-time marathon runners. By the end of their training the improvement in the state of their arteries was enough to make them appear four years younger.[1]

PVD is closely linked to other forms of arterial disease. About 60 per cent of PVD sufferers have concurrent coronary artery disease and 30 per cent have cerebrovascular disease[2] (see pages 110 and 121). Preventative measures for all these diseases are very similar. Regular exercise and high levels of physical fitness reduce three out of the four most important risk factors for PVD – that is to say, diabetes, high blood pressure and abnormal blood lipids. Regular exercisers rarely suffer from PVD.

A study of Japanese men has shown that both low fitness and muscular weakness predict an increased likelihood of erectile dysfunction.[3]

Exercise in the treatment of PVD

There are operations to restore blood supply – either bypass grafting or angioplasty (as for coronary artery disease but easier because you don't need to stop the heart) – but these are needed only when symptoms are severe or when the limb is threatened. The only other effective treatment is exercise, particularly walking. The best results are obtained when the sufferer walks to the greatest degree of calf pain tolerable for more than 30 minutes on three or more days per week for at least six months.[4] Supervised walking is more effective than unsupervised.[5] The Cochrane Review of this treatment covered 1,837 adults in 32 trials.[6] The treated groups showed significant increases in both pain-free walking distance and maximum walking distance.

The way in which walking improves intermittent claudication is probably by provoking muscle ischaemia (inadequate blood supply), which encourages the growth of new small blood vessels (collaterals) to bypass the narrowed or occluded arteries. Structural changes in the walking muscles also contribute to the improvement.[6]

Stroke

If you do an autopsy on an 85-year-old who died of a stroke, you will find five other things that person was about to die from.
S. Jay Olshansky, School of Public Health, Illinois

Atheroma ('hardening') can involve any artery in the body. When it attacks the arteries supplying the brain, the cerebral arteries, the result can be a stroke. Most strokes are caused by sudden blockage of a cerebral artery, depriving the part of the brain that it supplies of blood/oxygen/nutrition. There is rapid, irreversible loss of brain tissue, the most recognisable result being hemiplegia – one-sided paralysis or weakness. However, any region of the brain can be involved and result in such disparate damage as loss of speech, severe giddiness, changed behaviour, numbness, loss of sight and loss of cognition. Longer-term problems are often reported by stroke survivors one to five years after the stroke. The most common include poor mobility (58 per cent), fatigue (52 per cent), loss of concentration (45 per cent) and falls (44 per cent). Damage to the brain can be limited by rapid introduction of a stent into the damaged artery or by giving blood-clot-dissolving drugs – hence the public health campaign 'FAST' designed to promote rapid diagnosis and transfer to hospital.

According to the Stroke Association, there are more than 100,000 strokes in the UK each year and more than 1.2 million stroke survivors, many with severe ongoing disabilities. Stroke is the fourth biggest killer in the UK and costs the country about £26 billion annually.

Damage to the brain can be minor and repeated, and can result in 'vascular' dementia (see page 132).

Exercise in the prevention of stroke

As we have seen above, regular exercise reduces several of the factors that are known to be the most important provokers of strokes – obesity, high blood pressure, dyslipidaemia and type 2 diabetes (see pages 84, 95, 100 and 103). It would be impossible to carry out a long-term, large-scale randomised controlled trial of exercise for stroke prevention, but observational studies confirm that the incidence of stroke is between 20 per cent and 70 per cent lower in those who are physically active compared with those who are not.[1, 2] Moreover, these studies have shown that there is a dose-response relationship between the amount of exercise taken and the reduction in risk. That is to say, both duration and frequency of exercise are related to the reduction in risk – the longer you exercise and more often you do it, the more you reduce your stroke risk.

As you might expect, therefore, physical fitness is also closely related to stroke risk. For instance, slow walking pace in the over-65s carries an increased risk of stroke.[3] One study of over 16,000 healthy men showed a striking relationship between greater cardiorespiratory fitness and lower stroke mortality. Those in the high-fitness group had less than one third the risk of dying from stroke of those in the low-fitness group.[4] A study from the Cooper Institute in Dallas, Texas, followed 20,000 adults who had been fitness-tested and found a similar dose-response relationship between physical fitness and stroke risk – that is to say, the fitter the subject, the lower the risk.[5]

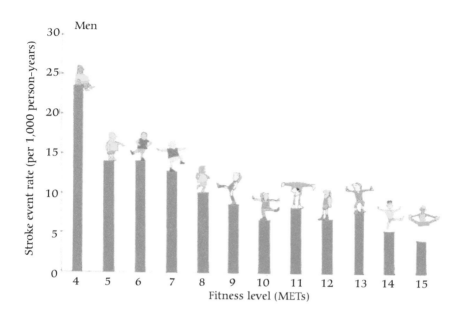

Stroke risk in men at different fitness levels

Exercise in the treatment of stroke

Exercise is vital to the restoration of muscle function. Rehabilitation after a stroke should start as soon as blood supply to the brain has been re-established to the best possible level. It is usually provided by inpatient physiotherapy, most likely to be in a specialist stroke rehabilitation ward. Treatment is focused on strengthening the weakened muscles to improve arm and leg function and restore mobility.[6] Balance exercises are an important part of this treatment.

There has been little research into the optimal frequency and duration of physiotherapy for post-stroke rehabilitation. What evidence there is indicates that more is better. Unfortunately, stroke rehabilitation is usually under-resourced, with patients seldom receiving adequate physiotherapy. Being in hospital is almost designed to reduce strength and mobility – 10 days in hospital is said to be equivalent to 10 years of ageing.

Hospital culture encourages lying and sitting rather than being active, driven by the desire to prevent falls in under-staffed wards: the sitting patient is less dangerous to him/herself than the mobile patient. Rehabilitation therefore has to be intense to overcome the de-training effects of being in hospital. Probably most of the gains are from the spontaneous recovery that is characteristic of strokes. The sooner the patient can be got home and returned to normal daily activities, the better.

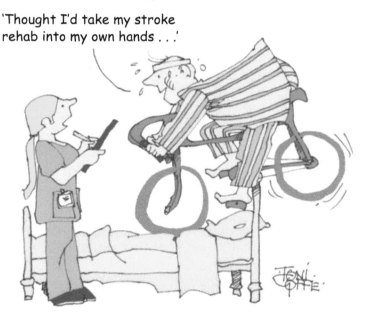

'Thought I'd take my stroke rehab into my own hands . . .'

A story of how it can be done

A model of stroke rehabilitation was provided by Roald Dahl. In 1965 his wife, actress Patricia Neal, had a disabling stroke caused by a brain haemorrhage. She was left with a severe speech impediment and one-sided weakness. Dahl feared she would become an 'enormous pink cabbage', so with his friends and neighbours he set up an intensive 6-hours-a-day regime of physical activity and speech retraining. Some professionals warned this was too much, but he ignored them. Pat was coached back to normality, 'slowly, insidiously and quite relentlessly'. She eventually resumed her acting career, even getting another Oscar nomination.

Long-term physical training

This hugely important part of the long-term care of the stroke patient is seldom applied. What a pity. A low level of physical fitness is one of the risk factors for stroke. Regular exercise reduces blood pressure, improves blood lipids, gives better diabetic control and helps with weight loss. A suitable regime has been suggested as 50 minutes or so of moderate-intensity exercise three or four times per week.

Other benefits of physical training

Post-stroke physical training has also been shown to reinforce the gains of early rehabilitation by further increasing cardiorespiratory fitness and muscle strength and improving walking capacity. Immobility, unilateral limb weakness, poor balance, cognitive impairment, reduced activities of daily living and quality of life, plus the risk of stroke recurrence all benefit. Greater self-confidence and independence are additional rewards, as are the amelioration of boredom and frustration.[7]

It is hard to overstate the multiple benefits of fitness training for stroke patients. It is just as effective as standard drug treatments, and maybe more effective in reducing the risk of recurrence and subsequent stroke-related death. The rationale for this is that decreased fitness is one of the risk factors for stroke and that, like other results of arterial disease, further episodes must be increased by failing to try to remedy this.[8]

A Cochrane Review has examined many of the problems faced by recovering stroke patients in a meta-analysis of 45 trials involving 2,188 subjects. The report concluded that cardiorespiratory training reduces disability after a stroke, improves the speed and tolerance of walking and probably improves balance.[9] Other studies have shown some benefit from exercise training for stroke victims, including improved cognitive function, self-confidence and independence.[10,11]

Parkinson's Disease

We may each have our own individual Parkinson's,
but we all share one thing in common. Hope.
Michael J. Fox

Parkinson's disease (PD) was originally described
as 'the shaking palsy' by James Parkinson in
1817. The main features of PD are stiffness,
difficulty with movements and a
characteristic so-called pill-rolling tremor.
Affected individuals have increasing
problems with physical activities such
as walking, writing and some social
functions, like holding a tea cup.

The prevalence of the condition is
about 1 in 600 in the over-65s, so with
an increasing population of older people
it is set to become more common. PD
progresses with age and may in time
completely incapacitate the sufferer.
Thought disorder and behavioural
problems may occur, and dementia is
common later in the disease. More
than one third of sufferers become
depressed.

Exercise in the prevention of Parkinson's disease

Only recently has evidence emerged that regular physical exercise
can reduce the risk of PD. A number of smaller studies had failed
to prove the link, but a meta-analysis of eight of these studies,
involving over half a million subjects, did confirm the relationship.
The review compared habitual exercise level with the risk of
developing PD and found that those in the highest exercise
category had 80 per cent the risk of PD compared with those in

the lowest category.[1] Furthermore, levels of physical fitness also predict the risk of PD and considerably strengthen the evidence for inactivity as a risk factor for the disease. A cohort of 7,347 US veterans were exercise-tested and followed up for up to 18 years. Men with high levels of physical fitness (VO_{2max} >42ml/min/kg) had only 25 per cent the risk for developing PD compared to those in the lowest fitness group (VO_{2max} <28).[2]

Exercise in the treatment of Parkinson's disease

Intensive exercise programmes have been shown to improve mobility and reduce disability in PD patients. A 2010 meta-analysis found that exercise, mainly physiotherapy, improves physical functioning and quality of life, leg strength, balance and walking in Parkinson's disease patients.[3] A more recent Cochrane Review of treadmill training in patients with PD found that this intervention does improve stride length and gait speed, although curiously does not improve walking distance.[4] Other benefits from exercise training have included improvements in various scales that measure severity of PD symptoms, and also improved balance, increased preferred walking speed and faster timed get-up-and-go tests.[5] Depression may be improved, as may be cognitive function and health-related quality of life.[6] An important finding of all these studies is the wide variability in response. Exercise can be very helpful to some, but by no means all, PD sufferers.

Several trials have tested different forms of exercise, including gait and balance training, progressive resistance training, treadmill exercise, strength training, aerobic exercise, and music and dancing.[7] Non-contact boxing is used in 871 sites across the world with some 43,500 participants.[8] Ping-pong also has its advocates.[9]

Finally, a word of caution. Parkinson's patients, with inherent balance problems, are vulnerable to falls sustained during exercise programmes. So far, however, this risk has not been shown to outweigh the benefits of regular exercise.

Psychological Ill Health

Mens sana in corpore sano. Juvenal, c. AD 100

Psychological illnesses are extremely common. The most frequent examples are depression and anxiety. A European study of depression found prevalence rates varying from 2.5 per cent in Santander to 17 per cent in Liverpool,[1] while a worldwide study found rates of up to 29.5 per cent.[2] Anxiety is almost as common, affecting as many as 16 per cent of the population over a lifetime. There is a plethora of other mental illnesses, but I will not be tackling them.

Why might exercise help?

One of the most effective and satisfying ways of combating stress is 'letting off steam', a process which usually involves exertion in one form or another. The release of endorphins mediates this feel-good rush. Indeed, the state of anxiety or emotional arousal prepares us for effort – the heart rate, blood pressure, blood sugar all rise, which was the natural response for our wild ancestors fighting for survival. Nowadays we seldom have the option of exerting ourselves when placed under stress – no way of dissipating the metabolic consequences of the 'fight or flight' response. We must sit and stew.

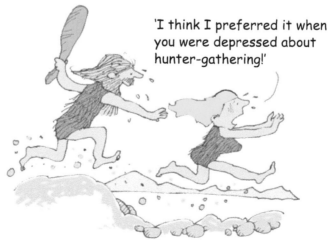

'I think I preferred it when you were depressed about hunter-gathering!'

Exercise in the prevention of psychological ill health

The preventative effects of exercise are more apparent for depression than for anxiety. A number of studies have indicated that regular exercise can reduce the risk of future depression. The most recent comes from a Norwegian study,[3] in which 34,000 people without either mental or physical illness were followed up for 11 years and their exercise habit compared with the risk of developing psychological symptoms. Undertaking regular leisure-time exercise was associated with reduced incidence of future depression but not anxiety. The majority of this protective effect occurred at low levels of exercise and was observed regardless of intensity. The findings suggested that about 12 per cent of future cases of depression could have been prevented if all participants had engaged in at least 1 hour of physical activity each week. A number of well-conducted studies have confirmed the definite, if modest, reduction in risk of depression in regular exercisers.[4-6] A 2012 meta-analysis of the association between regular exercise and subsequent depression included some 30 studies, 25 of which confirmed the association with a reduction in depression of between 8 and 67 per cent in those doing less than 150 minutes of exercise per week and 19–27 per cent in those doing more than 150 minutes.[7] A survey of more than a million adults in the USA found that people who said they took exercise experienced more than 50 per cent fewer days of poor mental health.[8] The effect was greatest in those with diagnosed depression and the optimal exercise dose was 45 minutes three to five times a week. Exercising more than 3 hours a day produced no further benefit.

A survey of 1.5 million people compared the type of exercise with its preventative effect.[9] The most successful approach was the combination of moderate to vigorous physical activity (MVPA) with muscle-strengthening exercise (MSE). At the higher levels (up to 300 minutes MVPA + 2 hours MSE per week), the reduction of risk of depression was about 40 per cent. An Australian study of 14,000 men confirmed that just meeting the recommendation for exercise decreased the risk of future depression, but that higher levels were even more effective (this did not include *extremely* high levels).[10] As might be expected, too much sedentary behaviour increases the chance of becoming depressed, particularly in young people.[11]

Regular exercise has also been found to reduce the risk of developing anxiety by about 25 per cent, agoraphobia by 58 per cent and post-traumatic stress disorder by 43 per cent.[12]

Finally, the effectiveness of physical activity is confirmed by the dose-response relationship between the level of cardiorespiratory fitness and the risk of becoming mentally unwell.[13] The fitter you are, the lower the risk.

Exercise in the treatment of psychological ill health

There is a general belief that physical activity and exercise have positive effects on mood and anxiety, and a great number of publications describe an association between physical activity and general well-being, improved mood and lessened anxiety. Some intervention studies describe exercise as lessening anxiety and depression in healthy subjects and patients. Recent well-controlled studies suggest that exercise training may be clinically effective, at least in major depression and panic disorder.

The Cochrane Review of the effect of exercise in the treatment of depression, involving some 1,356 participants, showed exercise to have a moderate clinical effect. The same report found that exercise also appeared to be as effective as either psychological therapies or anti-depressant drug treatment.[14] When targeted specifically at depressed adolescents, exercise also has a moderate effect.[15] Even light levels of exercise help,[16] but the response to exercise is related to the degree of increase in cardiorespiratory fitness achieved.[17] Exercise may also work for resistant depression which has failed to respond to other treatments.[18]

Although the evidence for positive effects of exercise and exercise training on depression and anxiety is growing, the clinical use, at least as an adjunct to established treatments like psychotherapy or medication, is still at a very early stage.[19] Exercise on its own, though clearly useful as an antidepressant, may not work so well as CBT (cognitive behavioural therapy).[20] The ideal is to use both together.

'Your recovery is remarkable.
What can possibly go wrong now?'

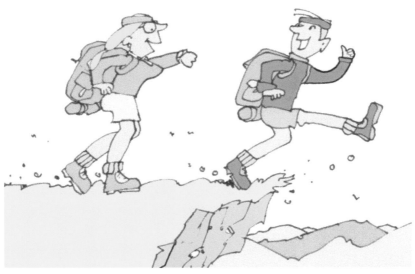

The Royal College of Psychiatrists recommends regular exercise as part of the treatment of anxiety and depression[21] and explains some possible reasons why it is beneficial:

Most people in the world have always had to keep active to get food, water and shelter. This involves a moderate level of activity and seems to make us feel good. We may be built – or 'hard wired' – to enjoy a certain amount of exercise. Harder exercise (perhaps needed to fight or flight from danger) seems to be linked to feelings of stress, perhaps because it is needed for escaping from danger.

• Exercise seems to have an effect on certain chemicals in the brain, like dopamine and serotonin. Brain cells use these chemicals to communicate with each other, so they affect your mood and thinking.

• Exercise can stimulate other chemicals in the brain called 'brain derived neurotrophic factors'. These help new brain cells to grow and develop. Moderate exercise seems to work better than vigorous exercise.

• Exercise seems to reduce harmful changes in the brain caused by stress.

Mental health

Just as physical health is much more than the absence of physical illness, so it is for mental health. There is a large number of instruments for assessing mental well-being from a variety of different perspectives:[22] emotional well-being, life satisfaction, optimism and hope, self-esteem, resilience and coping, spirituality, social functioning and emotional intelligence.

The Covid pandemic has highlighted the importance of mental health to the well-being of the population, with an emphasis on young people. The prevalence of poor mental health is higher in girls than boys and the level of physical activity seems to be the deciding factor.[23] Exercising for between 2.5 and 7.5 hours per week has been shown to be protective.[24, 25] In adults, there is also a relationship between physical activity and self-reported days of poor mental health, showing the more exercise taken, the less psychological ill health.[26] Active commuting – walking or cycling to work – helps, while sedentary time makes things worse.[27]

Dementia

My memory is not as sharp as it used to be.
Also my memory is not as sharp as it used to be. Anon.

Dementia is an advancing modern scourge and has recently been reported to have overtaken coronary heart disease as the most frequent cause of death for women in the UK. There are a number of different types of dementia. The two most common are Alzheimer's disease and vascular dementia, which between them make up

80 per cent of cases. About 47 million people in the world live with dementia and this number is projected to rise to about 130 million by 2050, while the figures for the UK are 850,000 rising to 2 million over that same period.[1] About 10 per cent of over-65s have dementia and a further 20 per cent suffer mild cognitive impairment. Over the past five years there has been a large rise in the number of people with dementia admitted to hospital as emergencies and many of them remain as inpatients for much longer than necessary because of lack of social-care support in the community. In 2017–18 there were 379,000 such admissions, up 35 per cent over five years, and 40,000 of these remained in hospital for between 1 and 12 months.

Curiously, for any particular age group dementia is getting less common, perhaps the result of the steady decline of vascular disease with less smoking and better treatment of raised blood pressure and lipid levels. However, this effect is overwhelmed by the steady increase in the age of the population, so demented people are becoming more numerous, though not as numerous as might be expected.

There are several known contributors to the development of dementia. These include smoking, hypertension, obesity and that cause of so much mischief – lack of exercise. About one third of dementia cases are attributable to these modifiable risk factors.

The devastation caused by this epidemic is hard to overstate – the ill effects are seen in every aspect of our lives. Most families will sooner or later have to face the emotional, financial and social problems brought by a relative with dementia. The cost to the health service and to social services of this rising tide of dependence is astronomical. The Alzheimer's Society has estimated that the cost to the nation is £24 billion annually, that by 2025 this will rise to £32.5 billion and by 2050 it could be costing the UK economy £59.4 billion at today's prices.[2] The economic impact of caring for each sufferer is currently some £28,500 per annum.

Exercise in the prevention of dementia

The evidence that dementia is delayed and reduced in severity by regular exercise is growing. Meta-analyses of all the prospective studies of the effects of midlife exercise have confirmed a significantly reduced risk of dementia and of milder forms of cognitive impairment in later life.

As an example, a recent study used the Swedish Twin Registry to identify 264 individuals with dementia who were compared with 2,870 unimpaired controls matched for age, sex and a number of other features. All were normal at baseline, mean age 49, and were followed up for an average of 30 years. Compared with those who did virtually no exercise, those who performed light exercise had less than half the risk of developing dementia, while those who performed moderate exercise had one third the risk.[3] A meta-analysis involving 164,000 subjects found a risk reduction of 28 per cent for dementia – and 55 per cent for Alzheimer's.[4] Higher levels of exercise are more protective and there is more evidence for the effectiveness of aerobic exercise than resistance training.

Higher levels of physical fitness in mid-life are also associated with lower risk of dementia in later life – those in the upper 20 per cent for fitness having two thirds the risk of dementia of those in the lowest 20 per cent in a long-term study of nearly 20,000 middle-aged Americans.[5] A number of studies have confirmed that having a high level of physical fitness delays the onset of dementia by around a decade. The Gothenburg Study of fitness and dementia included bicycle-exercise testing of 200 women aged 38–60 and followed them up for 44 years. By this time only 5 per cent of the fittest group had developed dementia compared with 32 per cent in the least fit group.[6] The importance of cardiorespiratory fitness (CRF) rather than self-reported physical-activity (PA) level was emphasised by a study of nearly 7,000 subjects which found that both CRF and PA are associated with quality of life over time, but only CRF was associated with preservation of cognitive function, particularly language ability, attention and processing speed.[7]

An overall healthy lifestyle does seem to be the best option for reducing the risk of developing dementia in old age and the more aspects of healthy behaviour the better. The Caerphilly Cohort Study looked at five different behaviours – exercise, maintaining normal weight, eating a healthy diet, not smoking and avoiding excess alcohol – and examined the rate of dementia over the following decades. Adhering to all five of these behaviours was associated with just one third the risk of dementia. You will not be surprised to hear that less than 1 per cent of subjects followed all five and only 5 per cent followed four out of the five behaviours. The biggest contributor to lowering the risk of dementia was regular exercise, which, on its own, reduced risk by about 60 per cent.[8]

The most recent and strongest evidence of the effect of exercise in preventing dementia comes in a meta-analysis of 39 trials of all forms of exercise – aerobic, strength training or a mixture of both.[9] For nearly 13,000 individuals aged 50 or more there was a clear benefit to cognitive function from taking the usually recommended level of exercise needed for health gain. The conclusion was: 'The findings suggest that an exercise programme with components of both aerobic and resistance-type training, of at least moderate intensity and at least 45 min per session, on as many days of the week as possible, is beneficial to cognitive function in adults aged more than 50 years'.

So far, so encouraging. However, a different approach to the evidence was taken by a large group from England and Scandinavia, who published their findings in the *British Medical Journal* in April 2019. They examined the individual participant data in more than 400,000 subjects from 19 studies, followed for an average of 15 years. They concluded that regular exercise had no protective effect against dementia![10] They did, however, find some protection for a sub-group suffering from dementia associated with conditions such as diabetes, hypertension and other causes of vascular dementia. It has been suggested that the apparent protection by exercise from dementia may be due to 'reverse causality' – i.e. the diminished physical activity observed before the onset of dementia might be due to a pre-clinical reduction in brain efficiency reducing the urge to exercise.

We view the subject of brain function through a glass and very darkly, but we do have a glimmer of an understanding of the possible mechanisms by which exercise mediates preservation of normal cognitive function. The region of the brain responsible for memory and spatial awareness is the hippocampus, which sits at the base of the brain. This area is one of the first to show loss of tissue in Alzheimer's disease and regular exercise in older subjects is associated with slowing the loss of substance of the hippocampus.[11] One year of aerobic exercise in a large RCT of seniors was associated with significantly larger hippocampal volumes and better spatial memory. Other RCTs in seniors have documented a reduction of age-related grey-matter volume loss with aerobic exercise.[12] Cross-sectional studies similarly reported significantly larger hippocampal or grey-matter volumes among physically fit seniors compared with unfit seniors.[13] Brain-cognitive networks studied with functional magnetic-resonance imaging display improved connectivity after 6–12 months of exercise. The ability of the brain to increase activity and functional nerve connections is known as neuroplasticity and this can be increased by bouts of exercise, the harder the exercise being, the greater the effect.[14] These studies support the belief

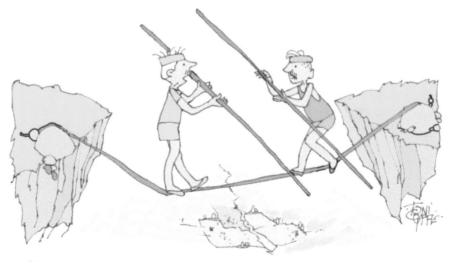

'We can't both be doing dementia balancing exercises . . . can we?'

that regular exercise can prevent dementia, but also suggest that physical activity could be effective for treating this otherwise pretty well untreatable condition. Both diabetes and obesity, conditions which are prevented by regular exercise, are associated with increased risk of dementia. This effect must play a part in reducing dementia in the physically active.

Exercise in the treatment of dementia

The hippocampus shrinks in late adulthood, leading to impaired memory and increased risk for dementia. Hippocampal volumes are larger in higher-fitness adults. A randomised controlled trial with 120 older adults found that aerobic exercise training increases the size of the anterior hippocampus, leading to improvements in spatial memory. Exercise training increased hippocampal volume by 2 per cent, effectively reversing age-related loss in volume by one to two years, leading to the possibility that exercise might reverse some of the effects of dementia.[15]

The 2015 Cochrane Review of trials of exercise as an intervention for dementia looked at 17 trials involving more than 1,000 patients. The main positive finding was that those treated with exercise were more capable of performing activities of daily living, but there was no evidence of improved cognitive function. The results, however, were very variable and the authors found the quality of the trials to be very low.[16] A 2018 review of the findings in 1,100 adults, average age 73, who had taken part in RCTs of exercise found that long-term exercise (at least 52 hours over six months) improved the brain's processing speeds in both healthy individuals and those with cognitive impairment.[17] Memory was not improved.

Subjects with mild cognitive impairment (MCI) have been shown to respond to aerobic exercise with an improvement in cognitive ability and a small improvement in memory.[18,19] The severity of the disease is probably relevant, and those with MCI seem to be more treatable than those with well-established dementia.

That is not to say that there are no benefits from exercise for more severely demented subjects. Such people can benefit from improvements in strength, balance, mobility, endurance and quality of life.[20, 21] A really important plus is improvement in activities of daily living, helping the individuals to maintain their independence.[22]

The management of dementia is a bleak and unrewarding field and we must do all in our power to prevent this disease. The most promising approach is regular exercise. Once dementia has set in, it seems that it may be too late for this to have much effect on cognitive ability, but there are still important quality-of-life gains for affected individuals.

Lung Disease

The secret of longevity is to keep breathing. Sophie Tucker

Lung disease encompasses a large collection of widely varying chest conditions. The commonest include chronic obstructive pulmonary disease (COPD – what used to be referred to as chronic bronchitis and/or emphysema), asthma and pulmonary fibrosis. They share the feature of causing more than usual breathlessness at levels of exertion that would normally be tolerated well.

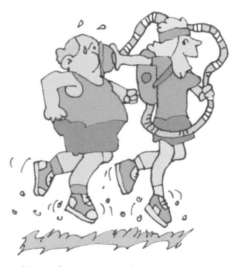

'It's the oxygen that makes this so easy for you!'

COPD is caused by a combination of progressive narrowing of the airways and loss of a proportion of the air sacs that make up the bulk of lung tissue. The main causes are cigarette smoking, asthma over many years and exposure to air pollution. There are more than a million people with COPD in the UK and each year there are about 30,000 deaths.

About 12 per cent of the population has been diagnosed with asthma. It is more common in children and young adults, but may continue into old age by when it has often morphed into COPD. There are about 1,200 deaths from asthma annually in the UK.

Pulmonary fibrosis is caused by progressive increases in fibrous (scarring) tissue in the lungs, interfering with the ability of the lungs to absorb the oxygen upon which we depend. It is a condition of later life, there are several different forms and the cause is often unknown. There are about 35,000 sufferers in the UK with an annual death toll of about 5,000.

Exercise and lung disease

There is no lung disease that is caused by or aggravated by lack of exercise (except when this has resulted in obesity), but any loss of lung function has effects which can be helped by being active and physically fit. When lung function is impaired, the supply of oxygen from the lungs to the blood is compromised. As explained in Chapter 4, lung function is not normally a limiting factor in exercise tolerance. The oxygen saturation of arterial blood is still high at maximal exercise. This is not true of exercise for patients with lung disease. As they increase the intensity or duration of exercise, the oxygen saturation of their blood falls progressively until breathlessness prevents further effort.

Exercise in the management of lung disease

Patients with chronic lung disease inevitably have low levels of physical fitness, a consequence of their limited exercise tolerance and their inability over a long period of time to take a lot of exercise. Pulmonary rehabilitation (PR) has developed over the past 20 or so years and aims to reverse this loss of fitness by providing a programme of graduated exercise within the limits of the patients' breathlessness. It works by increasing 'peripheral' fitness – more efficient blood flow to the working muscles and more efficient muscular performance. These changes allow better physical functioning despite the limited rate of oxygen provision.

PR has been shown to improve symptoms, give greater exercise tolerance and lengthen life for COPD patients.[1] A Cochrane systematic review of PR included 64 RCTs with 3,822 participants. The conclusions were that 'pulmonary rehabilitation relieves breathlessness and fatigue, improves emotional function and enhances the sense of control that individuals have over their condition. These improvements are moderately large and clinically significant. Rehabilitation serves as an important component of the management of COPD and is beneficial in improving health related quality of life and exercise capacity.'[2] The report found that hospital-based programmes were more effective than community programmes, but that the complexity of the intervention made no difference – it was just the exercise that did the business. PR works better if it is started as soon as possible after the episode of lung problem that initiated it. Among 2,700 COPD patients who started their PR programme within 30 days of an episode, the mortality at one year was 7.3 per cent compared with 19.6 per cent who started later or not at all.[3]

Patients with lung disease benefit from exercise but pulmonary rehabilitation programmes are underfunded, under-resourced and under-provided both in the UK and the USA. Also, NICE recommends PR for patients with COPD but not routinely for asthma or other lung diseases.[4] Fortunately, pulmonary patients can gain the considerable benefits of exercise from any source.

A questionnaire study of asthmatic patients found a correlation between control of symptoms and exercise frequency and intensity, improving from low to medium to high exercise loads but decreasing slightly for very high exercise loads.[5] Both aerobic and muscle strengthening are effective.[6]

Regular exercise does not reduce the risk of catching respiratory infections, but it does reduce the severity and duration of the resulting symptoms. Finally, regular exercise does protect against premature death from these conditions.[7]

Cancer

Cancer is a word not a sentence.
John Diamond, 1953–2001, journalist and cancer sufferer

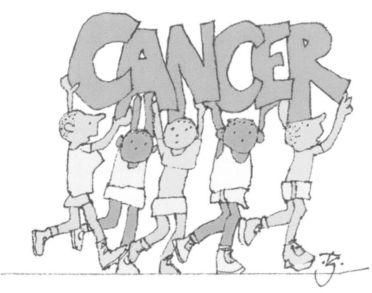

Cancers form a very large group of conditions that are extremely
common causes of disease, disability, suffering and death. Nearly 40
per cent of people will be diagnosed with one or another type of
cancer in their lifetime and cancer causes nearly 30 per cent of all
deaths in the UK. Cancers are also very disparate, varying from minor
skin excrescences to devastatingly fast-spreading and fatal
malignancies. The place of exercise in the prevention and management
of such a wide spread of conditions is likewise very variable.

Exercise in the prevention of cancer

It is not exactly clear why exercise prevents some cancers, but
there are several possibilities. These include reduction of
inflammation – a potent cause of a number of conditions – and
improved immune function with higher levels of natural
antioxidants. Whatever the reasons, it has been known for many

years that some cancers are more common in physically inactive people[1] and that the risk can be reduced by following the standard recommendation of about 30–60 minutes a day of moderate- to vigorous-intensity physical activity. Cancers involved include colon, breast, uterus, gullet, gall bladder, pancreas and kidney. Physically active men and women have about a 30–40 per cent reduction in the risk of developing colon cancer compared with inactive persons and there is a dose-response relation, with risk declining further at higher levels of physical activity. With breast cancer, physically active women have about a 20–30 per cent reduction in risk, compared with inactive women.[2] It appears that 30–60 minutes daily of moderate- to vigorous-intensity physical activity is needed to decrease the risk of breast cancer, and that there is likely a dose-response relation. Endometrial (the lining of the womb) cancer is also less common in physically active women by a factor of about 20 per cent.[3, 4] A large meta-analysis of 1.44 million individuals found that regular physical activity reduced the risk of 13 different cancers – by 10 per cent for the breast up to 42 per cent for the gullet.[5] Other cancers that were prevented by physical activity included liver, lung, kidney, stomach, womb, bone marrow (i.e. leukaemia), colon, rectum and bladder. The World Cancer Research Fund in 2009 estimated that 12 per cent of colon cancers, 12 per cent of breast cancers and 30 per cent of endometrial cancers in the UK are related to inadequate physical activity.[6]

As might be expected, there is also a relationship between cardiorespiratory fitness (CRF) and cancer risk. A low level of CRF has been found to increase cancer risk by up to 50 per cent and to have an even greater effect on cancer mortality,[7] reducing survival time free from cancer by as much as seven years.[8]

Mortality from cancer has also been linked to physical activity. A 17-year follow-up study of 480,000 adults related exercise mix to risk of dying from cancer and found the risk to be reduced by 30 per cent for aerobic exercise, 22 per cent for muscle strengthening and an amazing 50 per cent for the two combined.[9]

Closely related to lack of exercise, excess weight and obesity are among the commonest contributory causes of cancer. These include gullet, multiple myeloma, stomach, colon, rectum, biliary system, pancreas, breast, uterus, ovary and kidney.[10] Exercise clearly has a preventative role here. In 2013, an estimated 4.5 million deaths worldwide were caused by overweight and obesity; on the basis of recent estimates, the obesity-related cancer burden represents up to 9 per cent of the cancer burden among women in North America, Europe and the Middle East.[11] Body fatness and weight gain throughout the life course are largely determined by behaviour, including physical inactivity. Avoidance of weight gain has been shown to reduce the risk of cancers of the colon, gullet, kidney, breast and womb. Weight loss is even more effective.

An analysis of 180,000 women followed up for 10 years found that those who lost between 2kg and 4.5kg lowered their risk of developing breast cancer by 13 per cent, while those who lost more than 9kg lowered the risk by 26 per cent.[12]

The best current estimate is that around 1 per cent of all cancers in the UK may be related to physical inactivity (below a modest aspiration of 30 minutes five times per week), meaning that around 3,400 cases every year are linked to people doing less physical activity than outlined in government guidelines.

Exercise in the treatment of cancer

Prehabilitation

Prehab, for short, is the use of healthy lifestyle changes before embarking on treatment – in this case before surgery, chemotherapy, radiotherapy or all three. An exercise programme can improve the patient's general health, physical fitness and ability to withstand the rigours of the treatment regime. In the case of surgery for lung cancer, for instance, physical and pulmonary function can be substantially improved with a pre-surgery exercise programme, reducing the complications of the operation and recovery period.[13] Recovery is faster and more complete.

Rehabilitation

When it comes to the treatment of cancers, exercise is attracting increasing attention. Evidence is emerging to show that regular exercise can reduce recurrence of treated cancers after medical and surgical treatment, and can also prolong life. In one study of breast cancer, exercise treatment was associated with double the chance of survival over eight years and two thirds the chance of recurrence.[14]

Patients recovering from cancer and its management have to deal not only with the effects of the disease itself but also with the toxic effects of treatment, which can include pain, nausea, vomiting, fatigue, anorexia, anxiety and depression. Reduction in physical capacity, muscle strength and quality of life are very common aftermaths. An exercise programme can be the ideal antidote. A systematic review of the effects of exercise in breast-cancer patients found significant improvements in quality of life, cardiorespiratory fitness, physical functioning and fatigue.[15] A meta-analysis of trials of exercise treatment in a wide variety of cancer types concluded that such treatment led to improvements in quality of life and fitness both during and after treatment. The main benefit found for the active treatment was from moderate-intensity exercise but, after treatment, benefits had been derived from all forms of exercise. These include running, brisk walking, cycling, weightlifting, body-weight or elastic-band exercises, all of which can produce similar benefits. So far studies have not been designed to determine more exact exercise programmes for specific cancer types, nor the long-term effects of exercise: 'sufficient evidence is available to promote exercise to adults with cancer, and some evidence is available to promote exercise in a group or supervised setting and for a long period of time to improve quality of life and muscular and aerobic fitness'.[16]

Cochrane reliably sums up the benefits of exercise programmes for patients with cancer and concludes that exercise has beneficial effects at varying follow-up periods on health-related quality of life, with improvements in physical functioning, role function, social functioning and fatigue. Positive effects of exercise interventions are more pronounced with moderate- or vigorous-intensity than with mild-intensity exercise programmes.[17]

Osteoporosis

Some people get all the breaks. 'Get well soon' card

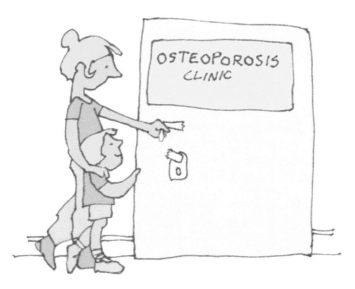

Osteoporosis is the loss of calcium from bone with consequent fragility and increased risk of fracture. We start to lose bone strength from the age of about 35 and the loss continues throughout life, but becomes more rapid in women after the menopause. From middle age we lose about 1 per cent of our bone mass annually. Some 3 million people in the UK have osteoporosis and they suffer more than 300,000 fragility fractures annually. These include such horrors as broken wrists and hips, leading to temporary or sometimes permanent dependency (see Chapter 11) and often to shortening of life. Ten per cent will die within a month and about 30 per cent within a year. Hip fractures alone occupy 1.3 million hospital bed days and cost the English economy £1.5 billion annually.[1] Post-menopausal women are particularly susceptible, though men are not immune.

Our bones are not inert struts to support our carcasses – they are living structures which continually renew themselves to maintain their functional strength, old bone continuously being replaced by new. Weight-bearing is needed to promote this process. Weightlessness, as in space flight, leads rapidly to loss of bone strength and osteoporosis.

Exercise in the prevention of osteoporosis

There are a number of ways of measuring bone strength, the most frequently used being bone mineral density (BMD). Logic says that the best way of preventing osteoporosis is weight-bearing exercise, particularly 'impact' exercise like running or skipping. Population studies involving athletes confirm this and indicate that high-impact sports, such as running, squash and weightlifting, lead to an increase in BMD, whereas low-impact sports such as swimming do not.[2]

An early start is important. The more time spent on moderate to vigorous physical activity in adolescence, the greater is bone mass by the age of 25. This is the age at which bone mass peaks and this is a marker of risk of osteoporosis later in life.[3]

For the spine and lower limbs, weight-bearing exercise is what does the business. However, the really important question is whether exercise reduces the risk of osteoporosis-related fractures, particularly of the hip or vertebrae, which can be so devastating for the sufferer. No intervention study has assessed the effect of exercise on the rate of osteoporotic fracture. That is to say, no one has carried out a randomised controlled trial of exercise versus no exercise to show that the exercised group has a lower long-term risk of fracture – such a trial would be extremely difficult to perform. However, observational epidemiological studies have indicated a strong protective effect. A study of 3,262 healthy men (mean age 44 years) followed for 21 years found that intense physical activity at the start of the study was associated with a reduced incidence of hip fracture, the risk being just 38 per cent of the risk for the non-exercisers.[4] Another study from the USA reported that women who had a high frequency of participation in outdoor sports had just 30 per cent the chance of suffering a hip fracture compared with those with a low frequency of participation.[5] A similar risk reduction has been reported in studies from Britain and Hong Kong. As one reviewer wrote: 'physical inactivity is currently proffered as the most salient explanatory factor for the increasingly high hip fracture rates reported by developing countries, as well as many first-world countries'.[6]

A neat way of showing the effect of exercise on BMD is to examine the effects on different limbs. Squash players from Finland showed a 15.6 per cent higher BMD at the proximal humerus (upper arm) of the racquet hand than the inactive arm.[7]

Cochrane in 2011 reviewed the evidence for the role of exercise in preventing osteoporosis and related fractures in post-menopausal women. They found a small but important reduction in osteoporosis from exercise programmes – resistance strength training being most effective in protecting the hip and combination exercise best for the spine. For the women studied, the overall fracture rate was 11 per 100 in those who did not exercise compared to 7 per 100 in those who did – a saving of 4 fractures for every 100 exercisers.[8]

One difficulty in interpreting this evidence is the confounding fact that regular exercise lessens the risk of falling (see page 152), so that fewer fractures may be the result of falling less rather than having stronger bones. Probably both are true.

Exercise in the treatment of osteoporosis

A definitive assessment of the effectiveness of exercise in treating osteoporosis was published in 2012. After analysis of 74 trials, the authors concluded that aerobic exercise and weight training do increase bone mass, or at the very least reduce the rate of bone loss, in osteoporotic (mostly post-menopausal) women. They found that the lower the BMD, the more effective was the exercise as a treatment. 'The best improvements seem to be achieved through strength training of high-loading intensities with 3 sessions per week and 2–3 sets per session.

Although significant effects can be observed after 4 or 6 months in some locations of the body, the efficacy of the training programme is greater when it extends for at least 1 year'.[9]

The National Osteoporosis Society produces a 60-page booklet of exercise advice for osteoporosis prevention and treatment (https://www.theros.org.uk).

– 11 –

Frailty

*We do not stop exercising because we grow old –
we grow old because we stop exercising.*
Kenneth Cooper, pioneer of aerobic exercise

Frailty in old age is a huge and growing problem, and the role of exercise in the prevention and treatment of frailty is one of the most important things I have to tell you about. This is an issue that affects all of us and decides the pattern not only of our futures but also of the social and financial health of the nation. The most important thing to understand is that frailty is **not** inevitable.

What is frailty?

Frailty has been defined as a 'clinically recognisable state of increased vulnerability resulting from aging-associated decline in reserve and function across multiple physiologic systems such that the ability to cope with every day or acute stressors is compromised'! In brief, it

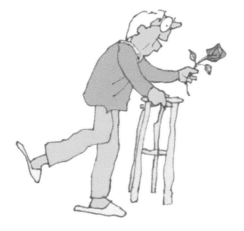
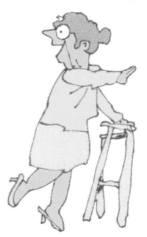

means getting old and feeble. Frailty is the condition of general weakness and debility that is often seen as an inevitable consequence of the ageing process. Some of the essential features include low grip-strength, low energy, slowed walking speed, low physical activity, and/or unintentional weight loss.[1]

Here is a test for frailty. Sit in an upright chair. Start your stopwatch, get up and walk 3 yards, turn round, return to your chair and sit down. A time of less than 10 seconds is normal, between 10 and 20 seconds is an indicator of encroaching frailty and more than 20 seconds is characteristic of frailty. Slightly more complicated is the five-repetition chair-rise test, which poses an increased risk of falling for those who take more than a minute to achieve the five up and downs. Walking speed is also an indicator of frailty – being capable of more than $1^3/_4$ mph rules out frailty; below $1^1/_2$ mph, the slower you are, the frailer you are likely to be. Among older people, those with a slow pace are three times more likely to need care than those who walk at faster speeds.[2]

What causes frailty?

Frailty is closely allied to loss of muscle tissue. As we age we all lose muscle mass and strength, a condition called *sarcopenia*. A degree of age-related sarcopenia is unavoidable, but the rate at which we lose muscle is largely dependent on how much exercise we take. By the seventh and eighth decade of life, skeletal muscle strength is decreased, on average, by 20–40 per cent for both men and women. Most of this loss of strength is caused by decreased muscle mass. The resulting progressive loss of muscle power leads to increasing disability and loss of independence. The prevalence of sarcopenia increases with each five-year age group, from about 15 per cent among 65–70-year-olds to as much as 50 per cent in over-85s and probably becoming increasingly common thereafter. It accelerates with the passing of the years.

As the age of the population grows, so will the numbers with sarcopenia.[3] The accelerated loss of aerobic capacity with advancing age has important clinical ramifications. The ability of older persons to function independently in the community

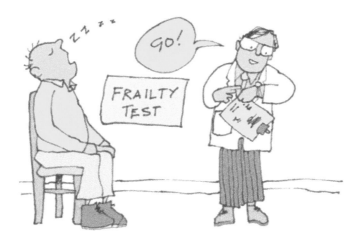

depends largely on their maintaining sufficient aerobic capacity and muscle strength to perform daily activities. The perceived degree of effort and breathlessness of a given activity is determined by its oxygen cost relative to a person's peak VO_2. People who have lost muscle strength tend to avoid tasks they think will require a lot of effort, setting off a vicious circle of further reduction in aerobic capacity, causing further avoidance of physical activity and further loss of muscle mass and strength.[4, 5] This is what frailty is all about – and it is **not** an inevitable consequence of ageing but, at least in part, a lifestyle choice.

The English National Fitness Survey[6] in 1994 highlighted the low level of fitness in the general population and the progressive further reduction with increasing age. Physical capacity becomes increasingly important as age increases. For 50-year-olds, not being as fit as they should be for that age will not make a substantial difference to their daily living (unless they are extremely unfit). But for an 80- or 90-year-old, poor fitness levels (relative to that age group) may mean that the individual is unable to maintain an independent life. The difference between being fit or unfit at this age means the difference between being able to get out of bed and dress unaided or relying on carers. Or the difference between being able to get up from a chair and put the kettle on or being dependent on others to do it for them. The level of VO_{2max} (physical fitness) that predicts loss of independence has been calculated at about 18ml/min/kg for men and 15ml/min/kg for women.[7] Personally, I believe that these figures are a deal higher than reflected by reality, but the point is well made that the lower your VO_{2max} the less able you are to look after yourself. Old people are particularly liable to become dependent if they develop an age-related disease (e.g. osteoarthritis). Frailty is usually the result of the accumulation of all the diseases discussed earlier – obesity, diabetes, heart disease, osteoporosis, osteoarthritis and general unfitness – and it is avoidable!

The consequences of frailty

The social and financial consequences of frailty are enormous and growing. When frail people become ill they have a higher risk of dying, becoming ill or disabled, or having to be taken into care than the non-frail and if discharged from hospital have a high rate of readmission – 40 per cent of frail people are readmitted within six months. If they need surgery, frail people are much more likely to suffer complications or die. Our hospitals are full of 'bed blockers' who needed admission only because they were frail and who are unable to go home because of lack of carers and lack of money to pay for them. The frail elderly occupy increasing numbers of beds in residential homes and nursing homes for dependent people. If able to stay at home, they require regular visits from informal or formal carers to allow them to keep a semblance of normal life. Frail elderly people are major users of emergency medical services, presenting with such problems as falls, immobility, incontinence and confusion. They are at particular risk of falling: 50 per cent of people aged over 80 fall at least once a year and about 5 per cent of these falls result in a fracture, most seriously of the neck or the femur (the hip). Falls are a major threat to older adults' quality of life, often causing a decline in their ability to care for themselves and to participate in physical and social activities. Fear of falling can lead to a further limiting of activity, independent of injury. Current estimates are that falls cost the NHS more than £2.3 billion per year.[8]

We have a growing army of dependent elderly people, with increasing social-care costs, increasing difficulty in finding enough younger carers and an inability to afford them. The trajectory of this problem is inexorably upwards, with the proportion of the population aged over 80 set to double over the next 40 years, while the number of over-85s requiring 24-hour care is also expected to double to 446,000, a staggering number. The media frequently publicise the crisis in social-care funding. The Institute for Fiscal Studies has predicted that, unless they are bailed out by the government, local councils will have to spend up to 60 per cent of their revenues on social care by 2034. The problems of caring for our ageing population will be compounded by cuts in funding and by the restriction of immigration on which staffing depends.

The role of unfitness in frailty

Frailty goes hand in hand with end-of-life dependence. The doctor and public health consultant Sir John Muir Grey has used a series of graphs (reinterpreted below) to illustrate the effect of physical fitness on ability to live independently.

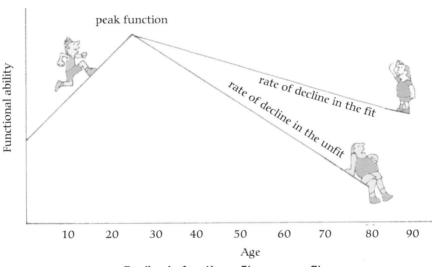

Decline in function – fit versus unfit

We all deteriorate in ability as we age but the fitter we keep ourselves, the slower that rate of decline, the flatter the trajectory of reducing function.[9] We can remain independent only if our ability is maintained above a certain level, shown on the graph below as the horizontal line. The less able we are, the earlier in life will we hit that line.

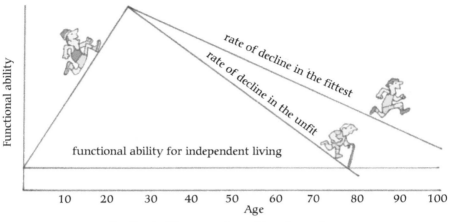

Decline in fitness and reaching dependence

Things get worse, because the frail elderly are particularly vulnerable to acute deterioration in health, mainly due to falls, fractures and infections. Such events lead to a sudden steepening of the curve of loss of function so that the line of dependency is reached much earlier (see below).

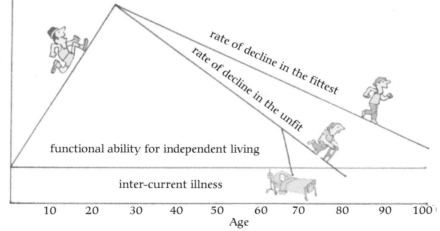

Accelerated decline in functional ability from acute injury/illness

And worse still is to come – hospitalisation. In hospital, immobility is the rule, a result both of the reason for admission and of the usual hospital culture of bed-rest for poorly patients. Unfortunately, the frail elderly not only start with reduced muscle mass and strength but also, when bed-rested, suffer a more rapid further loss than younger subjects.[10] For many this is the last straw in their goal of maintaining independence. They become stuck in hospital awaiting long-term care where that can be found. This disastrous progression of disability can be partly ameliorated by planned inpatient exercise programmes and these are now being implemented in many geriatric departments, with some success.[11]

Healthspan

The desirability of decreasing the period of dependency at the end of life cannot be overstated. We are living longer, but as our lives extend so also do the years of end-of-life dependency. What we should strive for is not just more years of life, but also more years of healthy and active life, which is sometimes referred to as 'healthspan' and is a much better measure of the health of the nation than lifespan. Shortening the proportion of our lives spent in end-of-life debility is sometimes called 'compression of morbidity'. This is what we need – to live well until as near to death as possible.

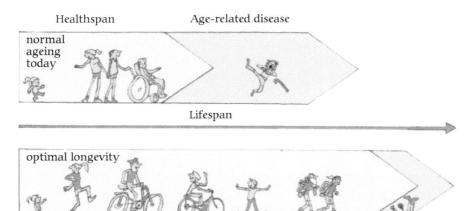

Healthspan and lifespan

Unfortunately, the most recent evidence indicates that, far from improving, our lives are worsening in this respect. The Office of National Statistics report in 2012 showed that a 65-year-old man could expect to be free from disability and long-term illness for a further 10.6 years, but by 2014 this had decreased to 10.3 years.[12] For women, the figures were 11.2 years falling to 10.9 years. Oh dear . . . Another way of looking at it is the life expectancy of someone born today. A boy born now can expect to live to the age of 78.5, but to have a healthy life expectancy (healthspan) of just 62.7 years – i.e. 20 per cent of his life will be spent with some form of disability or chronic illness. The picture for women is even worse – life expectancy 82.5 years, healthy life expectancy 63.9, giving a total of 23 per cent of life expectancy being lived with a chronic illness or disability. No wonder we have such a growing social-care crisis.

Exercise for prevention of frailty

Frailty is mainly the long-term result of an accumulation of one or more of the degenerative diseases described in Chapter 10. They are all promoted by lack of exercise and thus the main risk factor for the development of frailty is insufficient physical activity – over a very long period. The idle and the sedentary are those who are at risk. The key may be found in the difference between chronological age and physiological age. We are all aware of people who seem much younger than their real age would suggest – and increasingly of people who seem much older than their real age. This difference between chronological age (how long have we been around) and physiological age (how well can we perform) is measurable and enormous differences are apparent. In the FIT study in the US, nearly 60,000 subjects of all ages were assessed.[13] Fitness levels were used to assess physiological age and at each chronological age varied enormously – with discrepancies of between 18 and 38 years between chronological and physiological age. Physical fitness is a product of a number of factors, including age, hormonal changes, heredity, socioeconomic status, etc., but only one risk factor is easily influenced by the individual – the level of physical activity. A study of very active, non-elite, cyclists aged 55–79 found extremely high levels of fitness. For those aged 55 fitness was equivalent to the average for 20-year-olds, for those aged 65 it was equivalent to the average for 25-year-olds and for those aged 75 it was equivalent to 35-year-olds![14]

Similar findings resulted from the Stanford Arthritis Center study of runners aged over 50 compared with non-exercising controls, both groups being followed up for eight years. There were striking differences between the two groups in the development of disability, more marked in women than men.[15] In another study, over 500 members of a running club, aged 50 or more, were followed up over nine years and compared to a similar number of non-running members of the same community. The disability scores were low in both groups at the start of the study and remained so in the runners over the whole follow-up period. However, the disability scores in the non-runners rose steadily throughout the nine years. When this group was followed up for a total of 19 years the benefits sustained by the runners continued to accumulate.[16] The average time until the onset of measurable disability was 16 years later for the runners than for the controls. The health gap between the groups increased through the period of study and was still widening into the tenth decade of life.

The improved health status of elderly people who have exercised regularly has been emphasised by one study which found that the average 65-year-old can expect an additional 12.7 years of healthy life – meaning that he will live *disability-free* until age 77.7. Highly active 65-year-olds, however, have an additional 5.7 years of healthy life expectancy – they will remain disability-free until age 83.4.

Many other studies have confirmed that regular exercise reduces dependency in older people.[17,18] And an early start is important. The Whitehall Study initiated by Jerry Morris after his famous bus driver/conductor study (see pages 113–14) followed 6,357 civil servants for 20 years. Physical activity at age 50 predicted frailty at the age of 70 – those who were doing their 150 minutes' activity weekly at the start had the risk of future frailty reduced by a third.[19]

Frailty leads to 'terminal dependence', which is the interval between total independence and death. It is the idle and inactive who not only die earlier but also suffer a prolonged period of dependence at the end of life. Regular exercisers keep themselves fit, flexible and strong, and also reduce their chances of developing other diseases that contribute to frailty – heart disease, obesity, lower-limb arthritis, diabetes and dementia.

Exercise in the treatment of frailty

Although some improvements in function may result from exercise interventions to treat the elderly infirm, once frailty has set in it may be too late to make major differences to performance.

A 2008 meta-analysis of exercise interventions showed improvements in both functional and physical performance in the treated groups, but no increase in ability to perform activities of daily living (ADLs).[20] A further review in 2011 confirmed a limited benefit from applying exercise programmes to frail older adults and found that only more prolonged and vigorous exercise programmes were effective in improving functional ability – 'multicomponent training interventions, of long duration (≥5 months), performed three times per week, for 30–45 minutes per session, generally had superior outcomes than other exercise programs'.[21]

However, for elderly patients who already have some functional limitations, further decline in physical functioning can be slowed by maintaining even a low level of physical activity. The LIFE study in the US randomised a volunteer sample of 1,635 mildly impaired sedentary men and women aged between 70 and 89 years into a programme of physical training or no intervention. The treated group showed significantly better mobility after 2.6 years of training.[22] This effect is seen in 'younger' old people and the less disabled, but exercise may not help the very disabled, particularly those with severely limited mobility – exercise intervention is needed before debility has gone too far.

However, if it is to be any good at all, the exercise must be maintained – something that becomes increasingly difficult for the elderly. A trial that investigated weight training in nursing-home residents aged 90 years or older showed the training to be clearly beneficial in terms of strength and self-care scores – but the scores soon fell back to their pre-trial levels after the study ended.[23]

Balance and risk of falling

A particular role for exercise as a treatment for frailty is in the prevention of further falls in those who have already suffered accidental falls. Around one third of over-65s and half of over-80s fall at least once a year. Frailty predicts both falls and fractures.[24, 25] As we have seen (page 152), falls are the leading cause of death from injury in the over-70s, often leading to fractures – including 80,000 hip fractures per annum in the UK. The provision of exercise and education programmes to reduce the risk of falling is growing, an example being those set up by ambulance stations for the patients whom they have helped pick up from the floor. A large meta-analysis of such programmes involving more than 4,000 elderly fallers has shown subsequent reduction in falls of 30 per cent and in falls leading to fractures of 60 per cent – worthwhile indeed.[26] The 2018 Cochrane Review of the use of exercise to prevent recurrent falls in the elderly concluded that a combination of balance and functional training with strength training is effective.[27] If widely applied, this should reduce by a quarter the overall number of falls per year, which would amount to about 140 fewer falls per 1,000 older people over one year in the general population and twice as many in older people at high risk of falls.[28]

Conclusion

Frailty, a devastating condition of later life, is not inevitable and everyone has the opportunity to prevent it for themselves. It is never too late to take up exercise, but if you leave it too long you may have missed the boat as far as reduction in dependency is concerned. And as you get older it becomes increasingly important to maintain a physically active lifestyle. Lapsing into a lazy old age is a recipe for detraining and the onset of dependency.

– 12 –
Longevity

I'm not afraid to die, I just don't want to be there when it happens.
Woody Allen

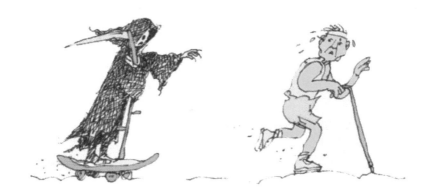

The bottom line – how long you live. There is no answer to the question 'What is normal life expectancy?' but it is certain that our population is nowhere near reaching it. The surprising fact is that, despite our thoroughly unhealthy lifestyles, until very recently we have seen a gradual increase in lifespan. In the years between 1991 and 2014 average life expectancy for men rose from 73.6 years to 79.4. For women the figures were 79.0 rising to 83.1.[1] This unexpected good news has recently hit the buffers, with figures produced by Public Health England suggesting that the trend has now flatlined.[2] Indeed, the Faculty of Actuaries has calculated that at the age of 65 the life expectancy of a man has fallen by four months and that of a woman has fallen by a whole year[3] – good news for the pensions industry, which will reap a reward of £27 billion in liabilities from company balance sheets.

The same is true in the US, where life expectancy fell in 2017 from 78.7 to 78.6, after rising from 69.9 over the previous six decades. More importantly, the duration of healthy life – healthspan – has been falling for several years, while the years spent in poor health have increased. We should not be surprised: just read on.

Effect of exercise on lifespan

As discussed in Chapter 7, there are two ways of judging how much a person exercises:

1. Assessing physical activity, either by questionnaire or by direct observation The former is biased by the individual's tendency to exaggerate, driven by so-called 'social desirability bias', and almost always gives a much greater exercise estimate than the latter. Direct observation produces the most accurate measure of physical activity but has a number of problems: it is difficult to do, difficult to compare between exercise types, requires special equipment and is expensive, and it gives a result that applies only to the period of observation. We can all up our game when we know we are being watched.

2. Measuring physical fitness There is a direct relationship between amount of exercise taken and physical fitness level, but with wide variations.[4] Other variables also affect the relationship, such as inherited characteristics. However, this method has the strength of producing a measurement that does not depend upon an unreliable witness – the participant.

Exercise volume and longevity

The most dramatic examples of the association between amount of exercise taken and longevity has been found in groups of people who take regular vigorous exercise as part of their daily life, be it either at work or at play. One such was Professor Jerry Morris's 1950s study looking at the fates of London bus drivers compared with conductors, which we have already considered in Chapter 10. The drivers were sitting for hours behind the wheel, unable to exercise. The conductors, on the other hand, were on their feet all day, moving up and down the stairs and getting plenty of exercise. Sure enough, the drivers had a higher mortality, largely due to a greater risk of coronary disease.[5]

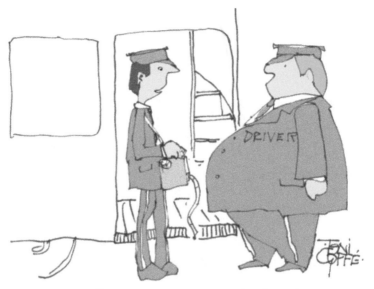

'Do you want to swap jobs for a bit?'

In those days the number of physically active workers was considerably greater than is the case nowadays – mechanisation has greatly reduced the role of jobs in making the working man take exercise. As we have seen, Morris repeated his findings in a comparison of the leisure-time activities of civil servants. Those who exercised vigorously in their spare time fared much better than their sedentary colleagues.[6] A very important finding was the presence of a threshold for the effect of exercise – it was only those taking vigorous exercise in their leisure time who benefited. Lower levels of exercise did not prolong life. An approximate level for this threshold was 40 minutes of exercise to a state of breathlessness three to four times per week.

These findings have been supported by the famous Framingham Study, which followed a large group of middle-aged and older citizens in the US. For this cohort, moderate activity increased the length of life by 1.3 years in men and by 1.5 years in women. High levels of physical activity further increased these figures to 3.7 and 3.5 years respectively.[7] A study of 15,000 Olympic medal-winners gives a different perspective, showing a total lifespan about three years longer than that of the general population – irrespective of the colour of the medal![8] Those involved in aerobic sport had better results than those who took part in power events, and the effect was also enhanced in those who maintained regular exercise after their days of Olympic glory, with an increase in life expectancy of up to five years.[9]

More recent examples of the life-prolonging effect of regular exercise have looked at those who take regular vigorous exercise as part of their sporting activities, such as runners, cyclists and swimmers. One study reviewed 500 runners, aged 50–59, and compared them with age-matched and sex-matched controls. After 19 years, 15 per cent of the runners but 34 per cent of the controls had died.[10] A review of all the available evidence indicates that runners have a 30–50 per cent reduced risk of mortality during follow-up and live approximately 3 years longer than non-runners.[11] Increasing the time spent running and increasing its intensity both produce benefit up to about 4 hours per week and a total dose of 50 MET hours per week. Above this dose of exertion, further benefit is doubtful and there might even be a small reduction of benefit. A much-quoted criticism of the benefit of exercise is the cynical suggestion that the amount of time spent exercising is about the same as the increase in lifespan. In this study, such cynicism is convincingly debunked. The authors calculate that every hour spent in exercise increases lifespan by seven hours! Not all studies have agreed on the optimal amount of exercise for prolonging life – some have found a ceiling effect,[12] but the majority have shown a clear association between increasing duration, intensity and frequency of exercise at least up to 300 minutes per week of vigorous exercise.[13–15]

Aerobic exercise is more effective for prolonging life than muscle strengthening, but a combination of the two has the greatest effect.[16] There is some evidence that regular swimming may be even more effective in postponing mortality.[17]

Look too at the effects of commuting to work. A study of more than half a million adults aged 40–69, followed up for five years, found that those who cycled to work had about half the risk of dying during this time as those who used public transport.[18]

These epidemiological studies involve long-term exercisers who have been at it for most of their adult lives. Is it ever too late to start? The answer is a qualified no, because the effect on longevity takes a while to kick in. It probably takes about 10 years of high levels of activity to increase longevity.[19] A cohort of more than 315,000 Americans aged 50–71 had their exercise habits tracked and were followed up for 20 years. Unsurprisingly, the mortality during follow-up was about 35 per cent lower in the habitually active group than in those who took little exercise. Surprising, however, was the finding that those who took up exercise later in life and then maintained it had a similar reduction in mortality.[20, 21] As *The Times* reported, 'It is never too late to get off the sofa and extend your life.'

Regular exercise, as we have seen, reduces the risk of a number of non-communicable diseases and this must largely explain its effect on life expectancy. However, there are other intriguing contributors, including an effect on cellular ageing. DNA is the genetic chromosome-carrying material found in all the cells in our bodies. Telomeres are the caps on the end of each strand of DNA and they protect the DNA from damage each time a cell reproduces itself. With time and repeated cell division, the telomeres become shortened and may indeed become so short that they can no longer protect the DNA, with subsequent cellular disruption. Telomere length is thus allied to cellular age and represents our biological age rather than our chronological age. Regular exercise has an effect on telomere length. There is a positive and significant relationship between cardiorespiratory fitness and telomere length, most marked in middle-aged and older people, which emphasises the importance of cardiorespiratory fitness for healthy ageing.[22] The reduction in cellular ageing has been found to be about nine years in very active older people.[23]

Physical fitness and longevity

There is a clear relationship between increasing habitual exercise and increasing physical fitness. For instance, running: every 30 minutes of running per week is associated with 0.5 MET higher fitness level. Numerous studies have confirmed the relationship between physical fitness and life expectancy – indeed physical fitness in middle age is the best predictor bar none of what age you will achieve, and that includes blood cholesterol, presence of obesity, high blood pressure, diabetes or even pre-existing heart disease, and cigarette smoking.[24] Only your current age is a better predictor of how many years are left to you. The reduction in mortality in the fit compared with the unfit is largely due to lower rates of cardiovascular disease and cancer.[25]

A summary of the results of 33 studies that compared physical fitness and mortality was published in 2009.[26] The population included over 100,000 people without heart disease, diabetes, high blood pressure or high blood cholesterol. The subjects had all had an initial exercise test to measure their fitness and were then followed for a mean of 11 years. Fitness was expressed in metabolic equivalents – METs (see page 30, 1 MET being the energy expenditure at rest or 3.5ml/min/kg) – and divided into three categories – low fitness being less than 7.9 METs (VO_2 = 27.6ml/min/kg), intermediate fitness between 7.9 and 10.6 METs (27.6–37.1ml/min/kg) and high fitness above 10.7 METs (37.4 ml/min/kg). There was a clear correlation between low fitness level and mortality – the risk of dying being 70 per cent higher in the low fitness group than in the high fitness group. Moreover, for every 1 MET increase in fitness (equivalent to an increase in walk/jog speed of 1km per hour) there was a 13 per cent decrease in the risk of dying. A similar study in 2015 found that the effect of fitness was even greater than this for younger age groups, with an 18 per cent lower mortality rate per 1 MET increase in fitness for those aged under 40, compared to the 12 per cent figure for those aged over 70.[27] A study from Cleveland, Ohio, tested the relationship between physical fitness and mortality in 122,000 people followed up for an average of eight years after a treadmill test. The relationship was stark, with cardiorespiratory fitness being related to lower mortality over the period of study. This was most obvious in those with the very highest levels of fitness – these individuals had just one fifth the risk of dying than the least fit. The greatest benefit between being fit and being very fit was found in the over-70s, confirming the effectiveness and importance of exercise in older people.[28]

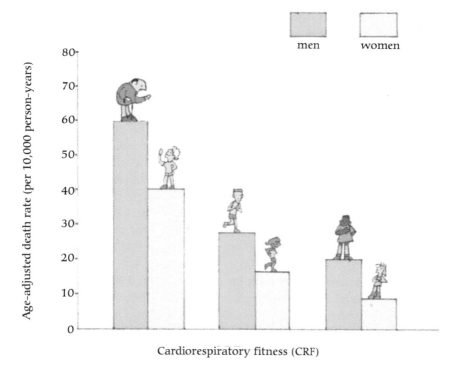

Physical fitness v. mortality

The Copenhagen study of middle-aged men put figures to the expected years of life gained at different levels of fitness.[29] More than 5,000 men aged around 50 had formal exercise testing. They were then followed up for 46 years. Compared with those in the bottom 5 per cent for cardiorespiratory fitness, those with low normal fitness lived an extra 2.1 years, those with high normal fitness lived an extra 2.9 years and the top 5 per cent lived an extra 4.9 years.

As with taking up exercise later in life, older individuals who improve their fitness also improve their life expectancy.[30] In a large epidemiological study involving older male veterans (65–92 years) with on average an eight-year follow-up, the lower the exercise capacity, the greater the risk of death. Mortality risk was 12 per cent lower for every 1 MET increase in exercise capacity, regardless of age – remarkably similar to the finding above. The biggest relative benefit was found for the higher fitness groups.

The facts are clear. Low levels of exercise and low physical fitness are both predictors of premature mortality and shortening of total lifespan. Low fitness levels have been calculated to account for 16 per cent of premature deaths, substantially more than any other risk factor, including cigarette smoking, diabetes, obesity, raised blood cholesterol and hypertension. And we should not be surprised that other measures of physical performance are also associated with longer life, including grip-strength, balance[31] and also leg-muscle strength.[32]

The Social and Economic Cost of Sloth

If we had a drug in our therapeutic armamentarium that conferred all the benefits of regular exercise it would be the single best treatment for preventing disease and improving overall health and life expectancy.
from 'Run for your life . . .'[1]

Maintaining good health and fighting disease and other health problems are enormously expensive. The NHS annual budget is set to be £212.1 billion in 2020/21, which is 9.9 per cent of GDP and 30 per cent of spending on public services. The social-care budget is even higher. NHS spending is planned to increase by 4 per cent per annum for the foreseeable future, but the demands are set to rise even more steeply. Currently about 18 per cent of the population is over 65 and this will have risen to 25 per cent by 2046. None of this takes in the astronomical costs of managing the Covid pandemic.

Increasing age brings increasing debility and this is compounded by medical advances which, while helping with the treatment of individual diseases, also results in longer survival and ultimately more cost to the NHS. Any effective treatment for the management of disease increases costs in the long term, because more people live longer with all the chronic diseases and dependency which old age brings. Exercise is the only treatment that does not increase NHS and social expense. By improving health overall and reducing old-age dependency, it actually reduces the bill.

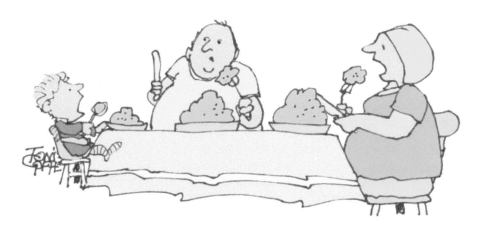

'Did you know you're costing the NHS
£149 billion a year?'

The cost of sedentary behaviour

Inactivity, or sedentary behaviour, is associated with poor health at all ages. The social and economic costs of this are impossible to calculate and the various estimates made by different bodies using assorted methods differ wildly – but they are all very large! One example calculated some of the associated costs in five common conditions which are in part caused by inactivity – cardiovascular disease, type 2 diabetes, cancer of the colon, cancer of the breast and cancer of the uterus.[2] They chose these conditions because they had well-validated measures of the 'population attributable fractions' for physical inactivity – i.e. what proportion of the cause of each disease could be blamed on sloth. For this small number of diseases – out of 20 possible conditions – their conclusion was that the cost to NHS-funding bodies was £800 million per annum. That sounds like a gross underestimate to me.

The medical costs of disease are only a very small part of the overall cost to the nation. For instance, the British Heart

Foundation and Oxford University used the same diseases to calculate the direct cost to the NHS.[3] They reckoned that in 2003–4, over 35,000 deaths could have been avoided if the population were physically active at the levels recommended by the UK government – and that physical inactivity was responsible for 3.1 per cent of morbidity and mortality in the UK, contributing over £1 billion to the direct health-cost burden to the NHS.

Again, this estimate vastly understates the overall costs to all those involved – the NHS, the national economy, the individual's finances and their employers' productivity and expenses. Some idea of the extent of these costs was given by another British Heart Foundation publication, 'Economic costs of physical inactivity',[4] based on 2010/11 figures. The table below illustrates the overall costs and the costs to the NHS of those conditions to which inactivity is a substantial contributor.

Condition	Cost to NHS	Percentage contribution of inactivity	Cost of inactivity
Coronary heart disease	£5 billion	10.5 per cent	£543 million
Type 2 diabetes	£1.2 billion	13 per cent	£158 million
Breast cancer	£0.3 billion	17.9 per cent	£54 million
Colon cancer	£3.5 billion	18.7 per cent	£65 million

For cardiovascular disease, there were almost 180,000 deaths and over 1.6 million inpatients (including consultant visits, ordinary admissions and day cases). The direct healthcare cost of all cardiovascular disease was £8.7 billion and the total economic cost (including healthcare cost, informal care and loss of productivity) was £18.9 billion. The average cost of a hospital admission for a CVD event is estimated to be £4,614.

For colorectal cancer, annual treatment costs were approximately £1.1 billion, 18 per cent of which could be prevented by regular exercise. The figures for breast cancer were a cost of £300 million, of which 18 per cent could be prevented.

For diabetes, the cost of direct NHS patient care (which includes treatment, intervention and complications) for those living with type 2 diabetes was estimated at £8.8 billion, and the indirect costs (such as loss of productivity) were estimated to be £13 billion, 13 per cent of which is preventable.

For obesity, the total annual cost to the NHS (including treatment and its consequences) was estimated to be £2 billion, with a total economic impact to the nation of around £10 billion.

A European perspective

A 2015 report from the Centre for Economic and Business Research calculated that physical inactivity was the fourth leading risk factor for global deaths and the cause of 500,000 deaths in the EU, with a cost of £84 billion a year to the European economy.[5] They reckoned that physical inactivity was a bigger risk to public health than smoking. The study also showed that being physically inactive goes beyond physical disorders. One in four Europeans (or 83 million people) is affected by mental ill health. The research estimates the indirect cost of inactivity-related mood and anxiety disorders to be over 23 billion euros a year.

The costs of care for the elderly

A new report from the All-Party Commission on Physical Activity estimates that inactivity is costing the UK £20 billion per year and causing 37,000 premature deaths. This financial estimate includes the costs of treating all those conditions that are caused by a sedentary lifestyle – obesity, high blood pressure, diabetes and all the others discussed above. It also includes lost working days due to sickness and lack of productivity of unfit workers. It must be a vast underestimate, since it does not take account of the huge costs of caring for elderly dependent people. A current estimate of the cost to the public purse of care of the elderly is about £22 billion – and the notional cost of informal care is an incredible £68 billion. Despite this, in the past five years £900 million has been cut from the UK Public Health grants given to local councils, who bear the brunt of the social-care expenses.

Inactivity also brings all the social costs discussed in previous chapters. The most important of these is the progressive loss of physical ability in later life – the difficulty in carrying out the activities of daily living, the loss of well-being, the loss of independence and the consequent financial burden of needing care. The overall benefits of good health are incalculable, but these benefits are there for the picking.

Political action is urgently needed to prioritise the promotion and encouragement of physical activity for the whole population, particularly in later life.

– 14 –
Encouraging Exercise

If your dog is fat, you're not getting enough exercise.
Anon.

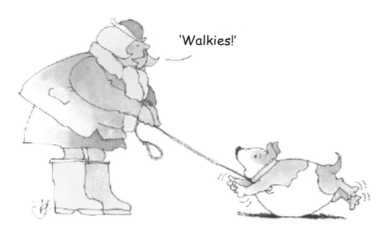

'Walkies!'

Every study of exercise behaviour confirms that the level of
physical activity in the population is lamentably low. The only
question is just how low. When exercise performance is
estimated from questionnaires, the level does not look too bad.
About 50 per cent of the adult population believe that they reach
the current government recommendation for physical activity.
(Later in life, the taking of exercise falls off badly – by the age of
75 the level is 8 per cent for men and 3 per cent for women). As
we saw in Chapter 7, however, when exercise level is actually
measured, the figures are startlingly different. The 2008 HSE
report, which did make measurements, found that just 6 per cent
of men and 4 per cent of women achieved the government's
recommended physical activity level – only one sixth of the level

of compliance indicated by individuals' own questionnaire response. As a society, we certainly need to put a great deal more money and effort into promoting exercise to a reluctant general public.[1]

Starting young

This book is primarily aimed at grown-ups – but the business of developing a national culture of exercise must begin in childhood. Unfortunately, children are as bad as adults in their reluctance to exercise. The Chief Medical Officer's guidelines recommend that all children and young people aged 5–17 should engage in at least 60 minutes of physical activity a day, of which 30 minutes should be in school. In reality, less than 20 per cent of kids meet this target and as they reach adolescence even this low figure plummets. Schemes to reverse the trend have nearly always been unsuccessful. A fun exercise programme aimed at maintaining physical activity into adolescence, GoActive, was trialled with over 1,500 youngsters in eight schools. At the end of the study, there was no difference in activity between the children in the GoActive arm compared with the controls.[2]

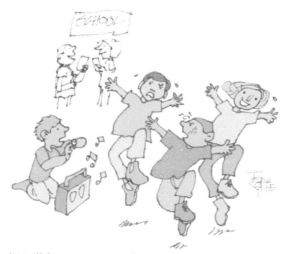

'We'll have to stop dancing soon –
we have to go to our school exercise class!'

The government does not help. The figures on school sports grounds are shocking. Since the London Olympics in 2012 the equivalent of one playing field per fortnight has been sold off and that rate has recently risen. In 2016, 21 schools sold their playing fields to developers, the highest number since 2013. Permission to sell was often denied by local authorities, who were then overruled by the Department of Education.

Schoolteachers, even if lacking their sports grounds, can play a big part in encouraging children to exercise outside school hours. One recent initiative has been the 'Daily Mile'. Participating primary schools – and at the time of writing there are more than 3,500 in the UK, with many more in other countries – get their charges to run for 15 minutes each morning before the start of lessons. Another promising area is the recruitment of internet technology. Over recent years there has been a surge of new online apps, blogs and videos specifically targeting young people with messages about personal improvement in their health and lifestyle. These technologies offer opportunities for young people, including collecting, tracking and sharing data – for instance about how far they walk or run. Despite their proliferation, there is currently no official assessment nor recommendation for their use, but there are great opportunities for applying IT in this field.

The most important people in promoting children's exercise, however, must be parents – maybe you, dear reader. The country is amazingly well endowed with altruistic adults, mostly parents, who supervise children's sporting activities – football, rugby, tennis, athletics – bravo to all of them. Parents may be helped by members of community groups who, in return, are allowed to use school playing fields (where these have been retained) in the holidays.

Grown-ups

In adult life the main bar to exercise is the lack of time resulting from gainful employment and/or bringing up kids. For you, the working person/parent, the most important incentive to exercise must be an understanding of just how vital this is to your future health, happiness and longevity. If you have not cottoned on to that by now, you have not been concentrating – start again and read more thoroughly!

The role of the medical profession

Encouraging people to take more exercise is a difficult task. Healthcare professionals should target appropriate patients, but seldom do so. A US study of consultations for diabetes or hypertension showed that exercise was recommended on only one sixth of occasions.[3] Even when advice is given it is largely ineffective.[4] A recent meta-analysis of trials of physical-activity promotion in primary care did find a slight increase in self-reported physical activity at 12 months, but those trials which also measured physical fitness showed no significant increase.[5]

There are many schemes that encourage GPs to prescribe exercise and most local authorities have systems for 'exercise on prescription' at their local sports centres.[6] The idea is that the GP 'prescribes' a course of exercise and the individual has an initial assessment at the sports centre, followed by a course of exercise of around 10 weeks at a cost somewhat lower than that charged to the general public. At the end of the course the individual is encouraged to continue to attend the sports centre at the usual rate. Exercise training and physical activity are not part of the usual medical student's curriculum, however, and this may explain why the level of referral to such schemes is extremely low. The uptake and completion of prescribed exercise programmes is even lower. Analysis of a number of these schemes shows that they do not lead to an increase in physical fitness, health-related quality of life or exercise habit in the longer term.[7, 8] The UK National Referral Database analysed 13 exercise referral schemes lasting between six weeks and three months involving 24,000 people. They found small improvements in the health and well-being of most participants, but these changes were too small to be clinically significant.[9]

The idea of exercise on prescription is a sound one, but more attention needs to be paid to barriers to attendance and continued adherence. Some of the factors that have been identified include poor organisation of the scheme, inconvenient opening hours, poor social support and exercise leaders lacking motivational skills.[10] However, regular telephone support and follow-up of absences for those who have been prescribed exercise programmes can be both effective and cost-effective in increasing long-term compliance.[11]

Prescribing exercise may not be part of the thinking of most general practitioners. However, GPs are extremely good at taking up opportunities to increase their income and this is the basis of the Quality Outcomes Framework (QOF) through which they are paid to achieve a number of clinical targets. If you think that your GP is taking more notice of his/her computer screen than of you, you are quite right. He is checking that he has made as much money as possible from you depending on your problems. He will be rewarded for including you on his obesity register, for getting your blood pressure or blood sugar to an acceptable level and for prescribing all the drugs that the NHS wants him to. He may be paid to refer you to various agencies for support and education – but there is no incentive at all for him to encourage you to take exercise. Perhaps if referral to an exercise programme were included in the QOF we might see a benefit for both the individual and the nation as a whole?

Encouraging the population to take exercise needs the commitment of doctors, who should regard exercise as a medicine, as effective a weapon against disease as any drug. The time may be coming for the lifestyle approach. As the *BMJ* put it, 'Is lifestyle medicine emerging as a new medical specialty?'[12] The British Society of Lifestyle Medicine was founded in 2016 and this approach is now being adopted by some medical schools, including Cambridge University. Ideally, lifestyle medicine should not need a label of its own but should become integral to the delivery of health care. In its delivery, the medical profession needs to be backed up by political action to make physical-activity promotion and facilitation key goals in their public-health strategy. It is also the duty of all health professionals to set a good example. Doctors don't smoke – they should also be seen to take exercise.

Enhancing exercise schemes

Exercise schemes can be somewhat effective, but only if combined with much input to encourage the individual and nurture the changed attitudes and behaviour which are required. A New Zealand study enrolled 1,089 women aged 40–74 into a controlled trial of exercise referral and achieved a modest increase in exercising rate in the treated groups at two years.[13] The intervention included initial motivational interviewing, regular follow-up telephone calls (a total of 75 minutes per patient) and a home visit at six months. Even with this level of input, the apparent increased exercise was not associated with improved clinical outcomes but unfortunately was associated with an increased risk of falls and injuries.

Other ideas

The British Heart Foundation (BHF) 2015 publication 'Physical Activity Statistics' includes a number of ideas for increasing physical activity in adults:[14]

• **Workplace interventions** Adults spend up to 60 per cent of their waking hours in the workplace, which should therefore be a useful place to start. Such initiatives include creating workplace exercise facilities, providing one-to-one exercise advice, encouraging the use of stairs rather than lifts, providing short breaks during the working day for employees to engage in physical activity. The Alberta Centre for Active Living (ACAL) in Canada has analysed some of the factors currently used to encourage increased physical activity in the workplace. They include challenges and competitions (pedometer challenges, physical activity and sedentary time), information and counselling (posters and handouts, individual and shared counselling), organisational (regular active breaks and moving about), the physical environment (office layout, active workstations, secure bike racks).[15] Again, the effects of these measures are limited. One multi-intervention health programme trial of 160 work sites did achieve an increase in self-reported physical activity at 18 months, but produced no change in any clinical outcomes such as blood pressure, blood cholesterol or BMI.[16]

• **Environmental interventions** Improving the environment in a number of ways can encourage exercise – walking and biking trails, outdoor gyms, traffic calming, encouraging 'active travel' – i.e. walking or cycling rather than taking the bus or train and notices promoting the use of stairs rather than lifts in public places. Residents living in neighbourhoods where it is easy and pleasant to walk have less likelihood of developing some health problems, such as pre-diabetes.[17] Evidence from existing low-traffic neighbourhoods is encouraging. The London Borough of Waltham Forest has implemented growing numbers of these neighbourhoods since 2015. A survey found that after three years residents had increased their walking by 115 minutes and cycling by 20 minutes per week relative to people living elsewhere in Outer London.[18]

In the United States, Active Living Research[19] has expanded the theme by specifying some of the environmental improvements that can encourage greater physical activity, including aesthetics of the area, plenty of vegetation, parks with open vistas, perceived safety from traffic and crime, general neatness, and play and exercise equipment. The importance of a good exercise environment was shown by the International Physical Activity and Environment Network.[20] Across 14 cities on five continents, the difference in physical activity between participants living in the most and the least activity-friendly neighbourhoods ranged from 68 minutes per week to 89 minutes per week.

• **Active commuting**, defined as walking or cycling to work, has been shown to be positively associated with physical fitness and also with lower BMI, obesity, blood pressure and insulin levels.[21] Active commuting reduces heart disease, cancer and age-related mortality, cycling being more effective than walking.[22] The bicycle-hire system in major cities (e.g. 'Boris Bikes' in London) has increased active travel. Sustrans (www.sustrans.com) is a charity which aims to enable and increase public exercise by walking, cycling and using public transport (which involves walking to and from bus stops, stations, etc.), leading to healthier, cheaper journeys. Their flagship project is the National Cycle Network, which has created over 14,000 miles of signed cycle routes throughout the UK, although about 70 per cent of the network is on previously existing, mostly minor roads where motor traffic will be encountered. On the downside, it is to be deplored that some train companies prevent the carriage of bicycles on commuter trains.

• **Community interventions** Social-support systems, group activities, buddy systems and 'Walking for Health' groups all promote more exercising, though to a limited degree. Telephone support and mass-media campaigns have their place.

• **Jogging and running** Another initiative has been the parkrun scheme – every Saturday morning some 300 parks around the country host 5km runs without charge. About 50,000 runners are out there each weekend. An excellent introduction to this form of exercise is the 'Couch to 5k' initiative, which helps anyone to get off the sofa and gradually increase their activity level to walking/walk-jogging/jogging 5k. The programme is supported by a website, a phone app and plenty of available encouraging and motivating podcasts.

• **Internet-delivered interventions** A number of schemes to increase physical activity within various populations have been delivered via the internet. This has the benefit of reaching a large number of individuals at a low cost relative to other types of intervention, such as making physical environmental changes or having regular direct contact with individuals. Internet-delivered interventions have produced positive results, but there is still insufficient evidence of their ability to produce long-term change. They have the particular advantages of providing easy self-monitoring and feedback information and enabling communication with health professionals or other users via email and chat. Many people find that feeding their accelerometer results on to a website allows them to follow their performance. Comparing it to that of others should be an effective incentive.

• **Smartphone apps** for encouraging exercise. Some concentrate on helping with behavioural change. Others measure activity, like the pedometer apps and the Public Health England app 'Active 10'. Results of exercise sessions, for instance runs, can be uploaded to a website which will track your performance and compare it with previous performances or compare you with other participants. The idea is that competition is a stimulus and should encourage you to keep exercising or even up your game. So far, there is little evidence of their efficacy in increasing exercise in either the short or the long term. One block to their implementation is the need for the user to be motivated to take exercise in the first instance. One hopeful development has been an app that is a game that demands physical activity. A randomised controlled trial of use of the game for 24 weeks in 36 type 2 diabetics found an increase in walking of 3,128 daily steps and increase in peak oxygen uptake of 1.9ml/min/kg – but, sadly, inadequate exercise and inadequate compliance led to no change in diabetic control.[23]

• **Pedometers** At an individual level, sedentary individuals can do much for themselves by just getting out of the chair and walking about for a few minutes every hour, going out for short walks, pacing about when answering the telephone. A pedometer or fitness tracker is an excellent addition to the armamentarium for encouraging increased exercise. Worn regularly, it provides the baseline and allows you to set targets that are easily monitored.

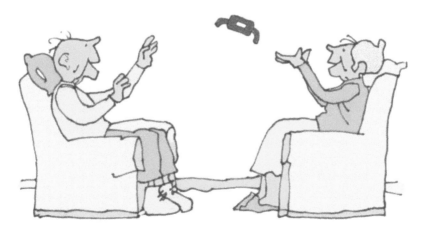

Pedometer exercise

Such 'trackers' come in a variety of forms with a variety of characteristics. They can monitor movement, calories burned, heart rate and even sleep patterns. The Consumers' Association produces a listing of available devices ranging in price from £18 to £700. If you decide that this is the right approach for you, choose one that is appropriate for the sport or activity you wish to track. Sadly, and grist to the mill of pedometer opponents, one controlled trial of weight-loss strategies found that overweight people using exercise trackers lost less weight over two years than their controls who did not use trackers![24]

• **Applying the concept of biological age** (see Chapter 7). It has been suggested that telling patients their biological age, particularly if it is much greater than their chronological age, could be a tool for encouraging them to become more active and thus bring the two ages into harmony.

• **Food labelling** to include the 'activity equivalent' of the calories about to be consumed. The results do not make very comfortable reading, which may be all to the good, provided it does not induce a sense of despair in the consumer. For instance, it takes a person of average weight about 26 minutes to walk off the calories in a can of fizzy drink. It takes a run of about 43 minutes to burn off a quarter of a large pizza[25] – oh dear . . .

• **Reducing exercise targets**, particularly for older people. The thinking is that for some folk even the rather modest goals set by the DoH and other national bodies may be a turn-off. Setting lower targets may help older sedentary people to move towards recommended activity levels – all exercise is good and a little is a lot better than none.[26] As a review by the National Institute for Health Research said: 'older people are more likely to keep active through structured group activities than exercising on their own at home. The social aspects of exercise and activity are particularly important. Successful approaches include walking programmes tailored to older people.'[27]

• **Walking** An analysis of the trials of physical-activity promotion in 1996 concluded that 'interventions that encourage walking and do not require attendance at a facility are most likely to lead to sustainable increases in overall physical activity. Brisk walking has the greatest potential for increasing overall activity levels of a sedentary population and meeting current public health recommendations.'[28]

For those who would promote exercise, nagging is not the answer, but gentle persuasion just might work, a bit. People need to be convinced of the joys of exercise. Choose an activity that you will enjoy and go for it. The feel-good effects will be surprising and the post-exercise glow has been described as 'on the orgasmic spectrum'.[29]

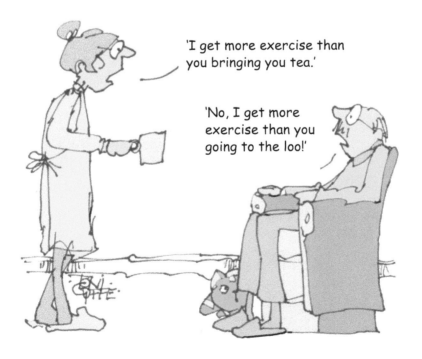

Ultimately, it is necessary to nudge people into exercise, remembering those motivating factors identified by the Allied Dunbar Fitness Survey. These were 'to feel in good shape physically', 'to improve or maintain health', 'to feel a sense of achievement' and 'to get outdoors'. Specifically for men were 'having fun' and 'relaxing', and for women 'looking good' and 'controlling body weight'. Remember also that many people are put off exercise because they do not regard themselves as 'sporty', because they are shy, feel overweight or lack energy.

The promotion of exercise in the community requires a politically led multidisciplinary approach strongly supported by the medical profession. Unfortunately, we do not yet know how this may best be implemented. Sport England, which was set up in 1994 with National Lottery money to do just this, has overseen a reduction rather than an increase in sports participation over the past few years. Now Sport England has joined with the Faculty of Sport and Exercise Medicine and Public Health England to launch a new project, 'Moving Medicine'. This aims to educate doctors and their patients to turn to exercise as the treatment of choice for many clinical problems and to introduce a culture of physical activity into the lives of us all. It is encouraging to see how many other organisations are involved in promoting exercise and producing policies to enable exercise to become the norm rather than the exception – the World Health Organization, the National Institute for Health and Care Excellence, the UK Health Forum, Sustrans, the Sport and Recreation Alliance, the Department of Transport, the Local Government Association, the Royal Society for Public Health, to mention just a few. My hope is that political actions and public education will produce a cultural shift that will make inactivity as unacceptable as cigarette smoking. To be effective, this needs to be supported by the full weight of public opinion and public pressure – though it will be difficult to tax it!

– 15 –
Sedentary Behaviour

My idea of exercise is a good brisk sit.
Phyllis Diller

'I'm more into aerobic dancing myself.'

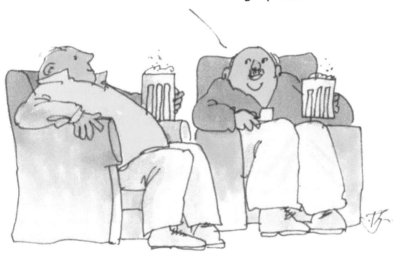

Sedentary behaviour is any time spent primarily sitting or lying down and which involves expenditure of 1.5 metabolic equivalents (METs) or less. Examples are sitting, watching television, playing video games, and using a computer.[1] Too much sitting, however, is distinct from too little exercise.[2] Just sitting about is dangerous in its own right even if you do take enough exercise. For adults who meet the minimal public health recommendations on physical activity on most days each week, the 9–10 hours of sitting that can occupy their remaining, 'non-exercise', time can still have a damaging effect on their health.[3] A new physical-activity grouping known as 'active couch potatoes' has emerged: those who apparently take the recommended amount of exercise but spend excess time just sitting around.

How much sitting about do we do?

The 2008 Health Survey for England (HSE) survey reported that around 40 per cent of adults spend 6 hours or more per day sitting down at weekends and slightly fewer on weekdays. A more recent assessment of sedentary behaviour comes from the HSE 2016. The self-reported average daily sitting time was 5.3 hours for men and 4.9 hours for women at weekends and 4.8 hours for men and 4.6 for women on weekdays. In each case, about 3 hours per day was spent watching TV. The trend was for more sedentary behaviour among the young (16–24 years), with an average sedentary time of 7 hours per day, and the old (70–79), at 9 hours per day – the so-called U-shaped curve. The figures from the US are similar. A national study of nearly 6,000 adults in 2015/16 found that 26 per cent sat for more than 8 hours per day, with 45 per cent not getting any moderate or vigorous exercise, and about 11 per cent sitting for more than 8 hours and being completely physically inactive.[4] Things may have got worse for young people with the huge growth in smartphone use. Among university students there is a direct relationship between time spent on the phone and decreasing levels of physical fitness.[5]

For the same age group, the influence of the Covid lockdown has produced some unexpected effects. In a study of 400 US college students, those participants who were not highly active before the pandemic actually increased physical activity after the closure of campus and the transition to remote learning.[6] The participants who were highly active before the pandemic, however, experienced a decrease in overall physical activity. Weird!

Older people were also considered by the SITLESS study, which examined the sedentary behaviour of 1,360 community-dwelling elderly adults, average age 75. It reported that 79 per cent of waking time was spent sitting, 18.6 per cent in light activity and just 2.6 per cent in moderately vigorous activity. Watching TV and reading accounted for 47 per cent of waking time.[7] There are clear occupational variations in sedentary behaviour, with office workers, as expected, spending more time sitting than blue-collar workers,[8] though office workers do partly compensate for this risk by taking more leisure-time moderate and vigorous exercise than manual workers.

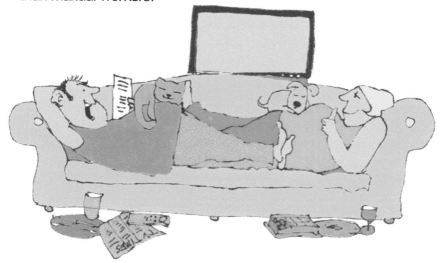

'Falling asleep while watching TV . . . we've lost 133 calories!'

The harmful effects of too much sitting

The risk of death increases for any sedentary time greater than 7 hours a day. One study of office workers found that those who exercised for one hour per day had a premature mortality of 6.8 per cent compared with those who did less than 5 minutes a day, whose premature mortality was 9.9 per cent. Both total sedentary time per day and length of sedentary bouts are predictors of premature death and the combination of the two triples the risk of premature mortality.[9] This has even received a label – 'the sedentary death syndrome'. The news is not all bad. Though regular exercise does not eliminate the perils induced by too much TV watching, it does reduce the impact. A meta-analysis involving more than 1 million souls found that you needed to watch television for more than 5 hours per day to reduce the benefits of a regular exercise habit.[10] About an hour's exercise a day offsets the ill effects of sitting at work for 8 hours.

The more you sit about, the higher your risk of developing cardiovascular disease and diabetes – independent of the amount of exercise you take when not sitting about.[11] The extent of the damage from sedentary behaviour has been quantified by a study conducted in Dallas, Texas, of the coronary calcium scores in heart patients. This score indicates the amount of calcium detectable in coronary arteries and is a good indicator of the presence of coronary narrowing, with its attendant risks of heart attacks and sudden death. For this group of over 2,000 patients, each hour of sedentary time per day on average was associated with a 14 per cent increase in coronary-artery calcification.[12] TV viewing time has also been under the microscope. For every additional hour per day of watching the gogglebox there is an increase in the risk of cardiovascular disease of 3 per cent and an increase in BMI of 0.54.[13] Other conditions that have been shown to be aggravated or even caused by too much sitting about include obesity and some cancers, while the death rate from all causes is increased.[14,15]

The cost of sedentary behaviour

Sedentary behaviour brings a substantial cost to the national purse. A Belfast study for the year 2016–17 estimated that the cost of sedentary behaviour to the NHS was £700 million per annum, with most of this due to the increased prevalence of CVD, type 2 diabetes, colon cancer, lung cancer and cancer of the uterus.[16]

Getting us off our backsides

How best to reduce sedentary behaviour, then? Perhaps surprisingly, fidgeting is very effective.[17] And there is no shortage of ideas given by the authors of the Dallas Heart Study paper: take a walk at lunchtime, pace about when on the phone, take the stairs not the lift, use a pedometer as a prompt to keep moving. Others have suggested using more 'active travel', such as cycling to work, getting off the bus a stop or two early, walking rather than driving for short trips, getting up and moving about during TV commercial breaks.

There is a move in some companies to introduce standing workstations in place of the traditional desk and chair. The Stand More At Work (SMArT) intervention is an approach adopted by one NHS trust.[18] However, standing instead of sitting may not be enough – and an active workstation has been invented. The Stir Kinetic M1 is a computerised desk which detects when its owner has been sitting for too long and moves up and down a few inches to force them to stand up. It can be programmed to account for the height of the user and the frequency of movement required – at just £2,000 surely a lifesaving snip!

– 16 –
The Complications of Exercise

The only exercise I take is acting as pall-bearer to my friends
who have indulged in strenuous exercise!
Anon., quoted in *Play Safe in Taking Physical Exercise*[1]

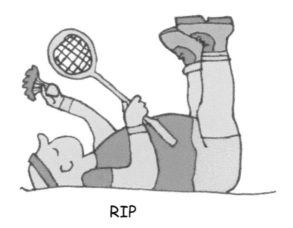

RIP

Despite the concerns expressed above, exercise is extremely safe – even strenuous and prolonged exercise rarely produces more than muscle or joint strains and sprains. Not exercising is far more dangerous than exercising. However, some complications are produced by any physical activity and I will start with the most significant (also the rarest) and work backwards.

Sudden death

The best-known, but also the rarest, complication of exercise is literally dropping dead. The incidence is about 1 per 50,000 in professional athletes in whom the usual cause is a congenital abnormality of the heart.[2] Sudden death is nearly always caused by a disturbance of heart rhythm known as ventricular fibrillation (VF). The muscle fibres of the main heart chambers, the ventricles, lose their rhythmic coordinated control, and each muscle fibre contracts and relaxes independently of all the other fibres. As a result, the ventricles stop pumping and death follows swiftly if normal heart rhythm is not restored. Definitive treatment is 'defibrillation', the application of an electric shock to the chest of the victim using a defibrillator. If a defibrillator is not immediately available, the victim can be kept alive by external cardiac massage until one can be acquired. Automatic external defibrillators (AEDs) are carried by all emergency ambulances and by many 'first responders'. They are also widely spread in community facilities and public places. It is not unreasonable for all concerned citizens to learn how to perform external cardiac massage and acquaint themselves with the way to use an AED – though, being automatic, the AED does make its use easy enough to allow completely untrained individuals to apply it successfully. St John Ambulance Brigades offer resuscitation courses across the country.

The most usual cause of VF in young people is an inherited abnormality of the heart – hypertrophic cardiomyopathy (HCM). This is inherited as an autosomal dominant gene, which means that on average half the offspring of a sufferer will have the condition. All the children of HCM patients should be screened and, if found to be positive, will usually be fitted with an implanted defibrillator which delivers a defibrillating shock if the heart goes into VF. It has been suggested that all professional sports people should be screened for HCM. Unfortunately, screening has a high false negative rate – six out of eight in one study of sudden death in young footballers had previously had normal screening results.[3] So screening is generally not thought to be a cost-effective endeavour and may also lead to a range of psychological, ethical and legal problems.[4]

In middle and later life sudden death from VF is usually caused by coronary heart disease, either at the onset of a heart attack or as a result of severe heart damage from previous heart attacks.

There is a widespread belief that sudden death from a heart attack is a result of 'massive' cardiac damage. In fact, VF is an electrical accident unrelated to the extent of cardiac injury. Those who are successfully resuscitated have the same prognosis as those who have not suffered this complication.

VF can be triggered by exercise – the rate of VF during competitive sports is about 1 per 130,000 person years;[5] during triathlons about one per 60,000[6] (mostly during the swimming section); and during marathon running about one per 50,000.[7] The risk of exercise-related VF in fit exercisers is far lower than in unfit non-exercisers. When the risk of sudden death during exercise is compared with the benefits of being a regular exerciser, the latter wins hands down. There is always a small risk with vigorous exercise, but the reduction in the death rate resulting from being physically fit easily outweighs the dangers of vigorous exercise.

Other cardiac arrhythmias

These include atrial fibrillation (AF), a very common condition of later life. AF is similar to VF but involving the 'ante-chambers' of the heart. Since the atria are not necessary for the heart to pump out blood, AF is not fatal, but it does reduce the heart's efficiency. The heart beats more rapidly and irregularly. The main complication is the development of blood clots in the atria. These can be dislodged and end up in the brain, causing a stroke. It is important that people with AF take blood thinners to prevent this.

AF affects about 7 in 100 people over the age of 65 and becomes gradually more common with increasing age. It is also related to physical fitness. The fitter you are the lower the risk,[8] except in those men who take excessive amounts of exercise. Above a level of about 1500 MET-mins (equivalent to about 5 hours of moderately vigorous exertion) per week, AF becomes more common.[9, 10] With appropriate management, this should not cause serious problems.

There is no good evidence that even very prolonged vigorous exercise is harmful to the heart.[11] Towards the end of very long bouts of exercise there may be some fall-off in the pumping action of the heart, so-called 'exercise-induced cardiac fatigue', but this reverses itself within 48 hours. Some electrocardiogram changes are also found in endurance athletes, such as evidence of a thicker than normal heart muscle wall, but again there is no evidence that this is harmful.

Other cardiac problems

It has been suggested that excessive exercise, particularly in older athletes, may damage heart muscle. Older athletes do have a higher prevalence of calcium in their coronary arteries, but this is not associated with an increased risk of heart attacks. One study of 'extreme exercise' examined 22,000 healthy men aged 40–80 and compared their activity levels with their risk of death during the period of study.[12] The most active men had half the risk of death of the least active, and those taking 8 or more hours per week at 10 METs or more were 23 per cent less likely to die than their less active peers.

Musculoskeletal injuries

Physically active adults (not necessarily older adults) tend to experience a higher incidence of leisure-time and sport-related injuries than their less active counterparts.[13] However, healthy adults who meet the usual governmental activity recommendations have an overall musculoskeletal injury rate that is not much different from that of inactive adults. Active men and women have a higher injury rate during sport and leisure-time activity, while inactive adults report more injuries during non-sport and non-leisure time. A possible reason for this lower injury incidence during non-leisure time is the increased fitness levels (endurance, strength, balance) of the more active adults. Inevitably, more vigorous exercise with its greater benefits does bring a higher risk of musculoskeletal injuries as the intensity and amount of activity increases. I would suggest to you that the benefits of a vigorous exercise regime greatly outweigh the temporary inconvenience and discomfort of these minor injuries. The common belief that it is exercise that causes chronic joint problems and osteoarthritis is bunkum – regular physical activity may even reduce the risk of developing painful osteoarthritis[14] by improving cartilage resilience and by increasing the strength of the muscles that support the joints. High levels of walking are associated with reduced need for hip-replacement surgery[15] and it has been suggested that cycling can also be an effective way of delaying hip surgery. Activities, such as jogging, that place greater strain on joints appear to be more protective than lower-impact activities and it is a myth that recreational running leads to osteoarthritis of the knees.[16]

It is probably true, however, that excessive exercise such as that taken by ultra-marathon runners and the like may bring an unacceptable level of injury.

Studies on injuries in adults aged 65 and over are scarce. The rate of injuries occurring during physical activity in advanced age, based on existing data, is very low compared to other ages. Based on current available research, there is no substantial evidence to justify the fear of getting injured through purposeful physical activity or in sports in advanced age.[17] Indeed, by strengthening bones and improving balance, the risk of injurious falls in the elderly is reduced by exercise training programmes.[18]

Stress fractures

These are small cracks in the bone, usually in the foot or lower leg, brought on by overuse and repetitive activity. High-impact or prolonged exercise are most often involved – running, football and basketball in particular. Sudden increase in activity or change in exercise pattern are causes. Other possible sites include the pelvis and vertebrae. The symptoms include pain and tenderness at the site of the injury. An X-ray may not initially show the fracture, but within a week the repair mechanisms can be seen. Treatment is rest and avoidance of further impact until healing has taken place – usually about 8 weeks.

Exercise and trauma

Some sports, like cycling, carry an increased risk of trauma, mainly at the hands (or machines) of other road users. Despite this, the cyclists are the ultimate winners. A study of 230,390 commuters identified 5,704 who travelled to work by bicycle. The cyclists were 3.4 times as likely to sustain transport-related injuries as the other travellers – but the overall mortality over the period of study was still lower in the cyclists.[19]

'This is great exercise for us, don't you think?'

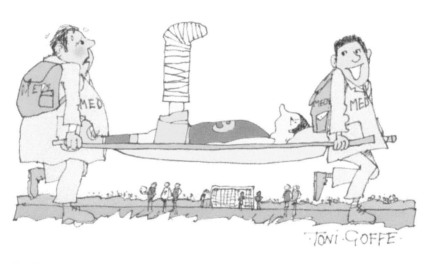

Contact sports often result in head injuries. Boxing is the obvious example, but football, rugby and American football can all involve repetitive head impacts which can eventually result in 'chronic traumatic encephalopathy'.[20] This causes brain damage and accounts for up to 15 per cent of cases of dementia. Another outcome is lowered testosterone production with resultant erectile dysfunction.[21] Wisely, the government has banned primary-school children in the UK from heading the ball in football training – but not in matches.

Extreme endurance exercise

Excessive physical activity does have complications. A number of cardiac indicators are worse in those undertaking very high levels of exercise, including enzymes released by heart-muscle damage and calcification of the coronary arteries.[22] None the less, high levels of physical activity and cardiorespiratory fitness are extremely protective against cardiovascular disease and cardiac mortality.

Other ill effects, found in sports students training for 5–7 hours per week, include increased bodily pain, sleep disorder and anxiety.[23]

Exercise addiction

People with exercise addiction experience loss of control to the extent that exercise becomes obligatory and excessive.[24] This is very similar to the obsession with exercise seen in some eating disorders, when the excessive exercise is part of the strategy to maintain weight control. Exercise addiction is not common, occurring in about 0.3 per cent of the general population and about 2 per cent of regular exercisers. In some sports it is much more common – up to about 25 per cent in runners.[25] It is seen about equally in men and women, though in women it is more often associated with eating disorders. Some of the characteristics include continuing to exercise despite injury and illness, and giving up social, occupational and family interests which might interfere with the exercise programme. Sufferers may report withdrawal effects when their exercise schedule is disrupted. The most effective treatment is probably cognitive behavioural therapy (CBT) with the aim not of stopping the subject from exercising but of helping them to recognise the addictive behaviour and adapt to a less rigid exercise routine.

Conclusions

If you have made it this far, well done you. If having read all this you have either increased your physical activity or have determined to do so, well done you *and* me!

Regular exercise is the most effective 'treatment' available for the prevention and treatment of a wide range of diseases, and for maintaining physical fitness, muscular strength and activity in old age – especially for improving quality of life. Indeed, a dose response between amount of exercise taken and quality of life has been demonstrated,[1] which means that the more active you are, the better your quality of life. In his Annual Report in 2009, England's Chief Medical Officer stated that the benefits of regular physical activity on health, longevity and well-being 'easily surpass the effectiveness of any drugs or other medical treatment'.[2] This fact is gradually dawning on the medical profession, but promoting exercise remains a major challenge in a world that seems to reduce or eliminate physical activity at every opportunity.

As we have seen in the preceding chapters, there is a dose response for the amount of exercise taken and the resulting beneficial effects – the more you do, the more you get out of it. Relatively speaking, however, the greatest return on your efforts comes from increasing from a low level of exercise to the next level up. In other words, the greatest relative benefit is gained by those who go from doing nothing to doing a bit (though the benefits are still well below those that can be attained by doing more). This is illustrated in the graph overleaf.

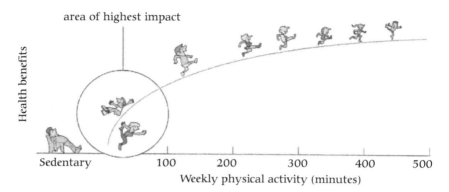

The incremental benefits of increasing fitness

The dose-response associations between total physical activity and risks of some cancers, diabetes and coronary heart disease have been assessed in a large meta-analysis. The quickest reductions in risk were achieved at between 600 MET minutes per week and 4,000 MET minutes per week, but this included all physical activities undertaken. Greater exercise doses had reducing impacts. While the greater the dose of exercise, the greater its effect, the less likely are the majority of people to maintain it.

The levels of exercise recommended by governments across the world reflect this reality. They are set at a level that has definite benefits but are not high enough to discourage most would-be exercisers from giving it a go. When it comes to exercise, horses are definitely for courses and vice-versa. So the message that I hope you will take from this book is this: if you do nothing, start doing a bit; if you do a bit, increase it a bit; and so on – and aim as high as is practical for you. Whatever it is that you do to increase your physical activity, be sure to make it something that you will enjoy or you will sooner or later fall by the wayside.

I would like to say that it is never too late to begin exercising. If it is maintained for a decade, taking up exercise later in life can become as effective as longer-term exercise.[3] However, the benefits of physical activity can only be gained by those who are physically able to do it and also able to continue it. Once disability has set in, taking up exercise is much less likely to do the business.[4] So don't put it off until it's too late.

Despite the known facts of the benefits of physical activity, less than 10 per cent of the population take enough regular exercise to improve their health. We need political action to achieve public awareness of these facts and to encourage everyone, and particularly older age groups, to increase their exercising habits. Perhaps the best target group would be the recently retired, who are young enough to be able to start exercising and have the time to do it. The gains will be great. Not only will they remain well, live longer and enjoy life more, but the period of ill health at the end of life will be reduced, with huge financial benefits for the whole population.

Glossary

Accelerometer Device worn to record movement, similar to a pedometer but providing information on other activities.

ADL Activities of daily living.

AED Automatic external defibrillator. Device which passes electric shock to the chest – used after sudden death in attempt to revive the victim.

Aerobic Requiring oxygen. Usually describing a type of exercise.

AF Atrial fibrillation – a common rhythm disturbance of the heart.

Anaerobic Not using oxygen. Usually describing a type of exercise.

Arteriovenous oxygen difference The difference between the oxygen content of arterial blood as it reaches its target and the oxygen content of the venous blood as it returns to the heart.

Atheroma Patchy narrowing of arteries, or 'hardening' of the arteries, responsible for heart attacks, strokes and peripheral vascular disease.

Blood doping Technique for increasing oxygen-carrying capacity of blood by transfusing an athlete with red blood cells previously extracted and stored. Illegal in competitive sport.

BMI Body mass index. The most popular way of assessing 'fatness' – by dividing weight in kilograms by height in metres squared.

Borg scale Also known as RPE, rate of perceived exertion. A way for exercisers to express how hard they find a particular exercise on a scale of 0 to 10.

Calorie A unit of energy. One calorie is the energy required to heat 1 millilitre water by 1 degree centigrade. One thousand calories is 1 kcal, sometimes written as a Calorie. This is the usual unit used to express the energy content of food.

Cardiac output The volume of blood pumped out by the heart in unit time, usually expressed as litres per minute.

CBT Cognitive behavioural therapy – a talking therapy for psychological problems such as anxiety or depression.

Cooper test A method for measuring physical fitness based on the distance that can be covered on foot in 12 minutes.

Diastolic pressure The lowest pressure reached in the arterial system between heartbeats. In a blood pressure reading it is the second figure, as in 120 over 80 (120/80).

Epidemiology The science of study of the causes of disease by association.

Gaussian curve The bell-shaped curve which shows the usual distribution of physical characteristics.

Glycogen A compound made up of multiple glucose molecules. Provides glucose storage and, when needed, is broken down into glucose for use in energy production.

Hippocampus A region of the brain concerned with memory and spatial awareness.

HCM Hypertrophic cardiomyopathy. An inherited abnormality of heart muscle which becomes abnormally thickened and is prone to causing dangerous disturbances of heart rhythm.

Joule A unit of energy. One kilojoule is approximately one quarter of a kilocalorie.

Lipoprotein A complex of protein and lipid circulating in the bloodstream, transporting fats around the body, including cholesterol.

Meta-analysis A summation of a number of different clinical trials to confirm or disprove the effectiveness of a treatment.

Metabolic equivalent, or MET The rate of energy production by an adult human at rest. It is equivalent to 3.5ml of oxygen per minute per kilogram of body weight (3.5ml/min/kg).

Mortality The death rate, usually expressed as the rate of death over a particular period or by a certain age. It is used to compare the effectiveness of treatments in lengthening or shortening life.

Myocardium Heart muscle.

Mitochondria Bundles of protein and enzymes inside cells. Their main function is energy production.

Q-Risk The risk of developing cardiovascular disease over the following years, expressed as a percentage.

Retinopathy Any disease of the retina of the eye. A particular feature of long-standing diabetes.

Sarcopenia Loss of muscle tissue. It is the most important element of frailty of old age.

Sleep apnoea Episodes of cessation of breathing while asleep. The typical sufferer is overweight and snores.

Stroke volume The volume of blood pumped out by the heart with each beat.

Sympathetic tone The background activity of the sympathetic nervous system, which controls such functions as heart rate and constriction of small arteries.

Systematic review A collection and summary of all the papers and research aiming to answer a particular question. When all the evidence is gathered the meta-analysis is the application of statistics to quantify the results.

Systolic pressure The highest pressure reached in the arterial system after contraction of the left ventricle. In the blood pressure reading it is the first figure, as in 120 over 80 (120/80).

T2DM Type 2 diabetes mellitus. This is the so-called maturity onset diabetes. The body still produces insulin but not in sufficient quantities to keep the blood sugar level under control.

VF Ventricular fibrillation. A disturbance in heart rhythm, with each individual muscle fibre of the ventricles (the pumping engine of the heart) contracting independently of the rest. The heart stops pumping blood and death ensues rapidly unless the heart can be restarted by defibrillation.

VO_2 The rate of use of oxygen by the body, expressed either as litres per minute or related to body weight as millilitres/minute/kilogram.

VO_{2max} The greatest rate at which the body can use oxygen to fuel maximal effort. This is the standard measure of physical fitness.

Watts A unit of energy expenditure (power) equivalent to 1 joule per second.

References

Chapter 1 A Very Brief History of Exercise

1. Boyd M, Eaton M, Shostak M, Konner M. *The Palaeolithic Prescription: a program of diet and exercise and a design for living*. Harper Collins, 1988

2. Juvenal. *Satire X*. c.AD 100

3. *The Economic Cost of Physical Inactivity in Europe*. ISCA Report, 2015

4. Fentem PH, Collins MF, Tuxworth W et al. *Allied Dunbar National Fitness Survey. Technical Report*. London: Sports Council, 1994

5. Church TS, Thomas DM, Tudor-Locke C et al. Trends over 5 Decades in U.S. Occupation-Related Physical Activity and Their Associations with Obesity. *PLoS One*, 2011. https://doi.org/10.1371/journal.pone.0019657

6. Paffenbarger RS, Morris JN, Haskell WL et al. An introduction to the journal of physical activity and health. *J Phys Activ Health*, 2004; 1:1–3

Chapter 2 The Muscles and Types of Exercise

1. Herbert RD, Gabriel M. Effects of stretching before and after exercise on muscle soreness and risk of injury: systematic review. *BMJ*, 2002; 325:468

2. Simic L, Aarabon N, Markovic G. Does pre-exercise static stretching inhibit maximal muscular performance? A meta-analytic review. *Scand J Med Sci Sports*, 2013; 23:131–48

Chapter 4 Exercise Dose: How Much Are You Doing?

1. Bushman, BA. How can I use METS to quantify the amount of aerobic exercise? *ACSM's Health & Fitness Journal*, 2012; 16:5–7

2. Ainsworth B, Haskell W, Whitt M. et al. Compendium of physical activities: an update of activity codes and MET intensities. *Med. Sci. Sports Exerc*, 2000; 32, No. 9, Suppl., S498–S516.

3. Mackenzie, B. *Energy Expenditure* [WWW]. 2002. Available from: https://www.brianmac.co.uk/energyexp.htm

Chapter 5 Physical Fitness:
the Best Measure of How Much Exercise You Can Do

1. Klausen K, Secher H, Clausen J. et al. Central and regional circulatory adaptations to one-leg training. *J Appl Physiol*, 1982; 52:976–83

2. Nanchen D. Resting heart rate: what is normal? *Heart*, 2017; 104:1076–85

3. Cooper, KH, A means of assessing maximal oxygen uptake. *JAMA*, 1968; 203:201–204

4. Fentem PH, Collins MF, Tuxworth W et al. *Allied Dunbar National Fitness Survey. Technical Report*. London: Sports Council, 1994

5. Health Survey for England, 2008: *Physical activity and fitness*. NHS, December 2009

6. *The Physical Fitness Specialist Certification Manual*. The Cooper Institute for Aerobics Research, Dallas TX; revised 1997. Printed in *Advance Fitness Assessment & Exercise Prescription*, 3rd edition, Vivian H. Heyward, 1998; p. 48

7. Fleg J, Morrell C, Bos A et al. Accelerated longitudinal decline of aerobic capacity in healthy older adults. *Circulation*, 2005; 112(5):674–82

8. Kokkinos P, Faselis C, Myers J et al. Age-Specific Exercise Capacity Threshold for Mortality Risk Assessment in Male Veterans. *Circulation*, 2014; 130:653–8

9. Rikli RE, Jones JJ Functional Fitness normative scores for community-residing older adults, ages 60–94. *J Ageing Phys Activity*, 1999; 7:162–81

10. Blaha MJ, Hung R. K, Dardarl Z et al. Age-dependent value of exercise capacity and derivation of fitness associated biologic age. *Heart*, 2016; 102:431–7

11. Fleg J, Morrell C, Bos A et al. Op. cit.

12. Pollock ML, Foster C, Knapp D et al. Effect of age and training on aerobic capacity and body composition of master athletes. *J. Appl. Physiol*, 1987; 62:725–7

13. Rogers MA, Hagberg JM, Martin WH et al. Decline in VO_{2max} with aging in master athletes and sedentary men. *J Appl Physiol*, 1990; 68:2195–9

Chapter 6 How Often, How Hard and How Long?

1. Department of Health and Social Care. *UK Chief Medical Officer's Physical Activities Guideline*. September 2019

2. Piercy KL, Troiana RP, Ballard RM et al. The physical activity guideline for Americans. *JAMA*, 20 November 2018; 320(19):2020–28. Doi: 10.1001/jama.2018.14854

3. Sparling PB, Howard BJ, Dunstan DW et al. Recommendations for physical activity in older adults. *BMJ*, 21 January 2015; 350:h100

Chapter 7 How Much Exercise Do We *Really* Take?

1. The Health Survey for England, 2008: *Physical Activity and Fitness*. Health and Social Care Information Centre, 2009. www.hscic.gov.uk/pubs/hse08physicalactivity

2. activepeople.sportengland.org/; 2021

3. www.gov.uk/government/collections/national-travel-surveystatistics; 2021

4. data.gov.uk/dataset/general_household_survey; 2021

5. https://www.gov.uk/government/publications/uk-physical-activity-guidelines. 2011

6. The Health Survey for England, 2012: *Physical Activity*. Health and Social Care Information Centre, 2013. www.hscic.gov.uk/pubs/hse12physicalactivity

7. Health Survey for England, 2016: *Physical Activity in Adults*. Health and Social Care Information Centre, 2017. www.hscic.gov.uk/pubs/hse16physicalactivity

8. Talbot A, Morrell C, Metter E, Fleg J. Comparison of cardiorespiratory fitness versus leisure time physical activity as predictors of coronary events in men aged ≤65 years and >65 years. *Am J Cardiol*, 2002; 89:1187–92

Chapter 8 So Just How Fit Are We?

1. Fentem PH, Collins MF, Tuxworth W et al. *Allied Dunbar National Fitness Survey. Technical Report*. London: Sports Council, 1994

2. The Health Survey for England, 2008: *Physical Activity and Fitness*. Health and Social Care Information Centre, 2009. www.hscic.gov.uk/pubs/hse08physicalactivity

Chapter 9 Evidence: Interpreting the Science

1. *Boundless Microbiology*: Epidemiology. Lumen Learning, 2021. www.courses.lumenlearning.com/boundless-microgbiology/chapter/principles-of-epidmiology/

2. Lundh A, Lexchin J, Mintzes J et al. Industry sponsorship and research outcomes. Cochrane Database of Systematic Reviews, 2017

Chapter 10 Exercise, Fitness and Disease: How They All Relate

Obesity

1. Global BMI Mortality Collaboration. Body-mass index and all-cause mortality: individual-participant-data meta-analysis of 239 prospective studies in four continents. *Lancet*, 2016; 388:776–86

2. Bray GA. Obesity: historical development of scientific and cultural ideas. *Int J Obes*, 1990; 14:909–26

3. Nuffield Trust. https://www.nuffieldtrust.org.uk/resource/obesity

4. Shaw KA, Gennat HC, O'Rourke P, Del Mar C. Exercise for overweight or obesity. Cochrane Database of Systematic Reviews, 2006; Issue 4. Art. No. CD003817. Doi: 10.1002/14651858.CD003817.pub3

5. Griffith R, Lluberas R, Luhrmann M. Gluttony and sloth? Calories, labor market activity and the rise of obesity. *J Europ Econom Assoc*, 2016; 14:1253–86

6. DEFRA. *Detailed annual statistics on family food and drink purchases*. 2013. www.gov.uk/government/statistical-data-sets/family-food-datasets

7. The Obesity Health Alliance. obesityhealthalliance.org.uk

8. Bailey R. Evaluating calorie intake. February 2018. https://datasciencecampus.ons.gov.uk/eclipse/

9. Guo W, Key TJ, Reeves GK. Accelerometer compared with questionnaire measures of physical activity in relation to body size and composition: a large cross-sectional analysis of UK Biobank. *BMJ Open*, 2019; 9:e024206. Doi: 10.1136/bmjopen-2018-024206

10. Tan M, He F, MacGregor G. Obesity and covid-19: The role of the food industry: The viral pandemic makes tackling the obesity pandemic even more urgent. *BMJ*, 2020; 369:m2237. http://dx.doi.org/10.1136/bmj.m2237

11. Somoes EJ, Kobau R, Kapp J et al. Associations of physical activity and body mass index with activities of daily living in older adults. *J Commun Health*, 2006; 31:453–67

12. Prospective Studies Collaboration. Body-mass index and cause-specific mortality in 900,000 adults: collaborative analyses of 57 prospective studies. *Lancet*, 2009; 373:1083–96

13. Ranjbar N, Turner L, Wanklyn P. Obesity – the deadly disease no one dies of. ECOICO, 2020. Poster.

14. Global BMI Mortality Collaboration. Op. cit.

15. Aune D, Sen A, Prasad M et al. Body mass index and mortality: patterns and paradoxes. *BMJ*, 2016; 353:i2156

16. Wareham NJ, van Sluijs EMF, Ekelund U. Physical activity and obesity prevention: a review of the current evidence. *Proc Nutr Soc*, 2005; 64:229–47

17. Slenz CA, Duscha BD, Johnson JL et al. Effects of the amount of exercise on body weight, body composition and measures of central obesity. *Arch Int Med*, 2004; 164:31–9

18. Shaw KA, Gennat HC, O'Rourke P, Del Mar C. Op. cit.

19. Hu FB, Willett WC, Li et al. Adiposity as compared with physical activity in predicting mortality among women. *N Eng J Med*, 2004; 351:2694–703

20. Verheggen RJHM, Maessen MFH, Green DJ et al. A systematic review and meta-analysis on the effects of exercise training versus hypocaloric diet: distinct effects on body weight and visceral adipose tissue. *Obesity Reviews*, 2016; 17: 664–90

21. Sui X, LaMonte MJ, Laditka JN et al. Cardiorespiratory fitness and adiposity as mortality predictors in older adults. *JAMA*, 2007; 298:2507–16

22. Obesity and fitness, Briefing paper. Public Health England, October 2014

23. Viana RB, Naves JPA, Coswig VS et al. Is interval training the magic bullet for fat loss? A systematic review and meta-analysis comparing moderate-intensity continuous training with high-intensity interval training (HIIT). *British Journal of Sports Medicine*, 2019; 53:655–64

24. John M. Jakicic, PhD; Bess H. Marcus, PhD; Wei Lang, PhD; et al. Effect of exercise on 24-month weight loss maintenance in overweight women. *Arch Intern Med*, 2008; 198:1550–59

25. Ostendorf DM, Caldwell AE, Creasy SA et al. Physical activity energy expenditure and total daily energy expenditure in successful weight loss maintainers. *Obesity*, 2018; 27:496–504

Raised blood pressure (hypertension)

1. The SPRINT Research Group. A Randomized Trial of Intensive versus Standard Blood-Pressure Control. *N Engl J Med*, 2015; 373:2103–16

2. Masoli J, Delgado J, Pilling L et al. Blood pressure in frail older adults: associations with cardiovascular outcomes and all-cause mortality. *Age Ageing*, 24 August 2020; 49(5):807–13. Doi: 10.1093/ageing/afaa028

3. Pajewski NM, Berlowitz DR, Bress AP et al. Intensive vs Standard Blood Pressure Control in Adults 80 Years or Older: A Secondary Analysis of the Systolic Blood Pressure Intervention Trial. *J Am Geriatr Soc*, March 2020; 68(3):496–504. Doi: 10.1111/jgs.16272

4. Gillespie CD, Hurvitz KA. Prevalence of Hypertension and Controlled Hypertension – United States, 2007–2010. Centers for Disease Control and Prevention Supplements, 22 November 2013 /62(03); 144–48

5. Lawes CM, Vander Hoorn S, Rodgers A. International Society of Hypertension: Global burden of blood-pressure-related disease, 2001. *Lancet*, 2008; 371:1513

6. Paffenbarger RS Jr, Wing AL, Hyde RT, Jung DL. Physical activity and incidence of hypertension in college alumni. *Amer J Epidemiol*, March 1983; 117(3):245–57

7. Gyntelberg F, Meyer J. Relationship between blood pressure and physical fitness, smoking and alcohol consumption in Copenhagen males aged 40–59. *Acta Med Scand*, Vol. 1974; 195:375–80

8. Mielki G, Bailey T, Burton N, Brown WJ. Participation in sports/recreational activities and incidence of hypertension, diabetes and obesity in adults. *Scandinavian Journal of Medicine & Science in Sports*, August 2020

9. Bennie JA, Lee DC, Brellenthin AG, De Cocker K. Muscle-strengthening exercise and prevalent hypertension among 1.5 million adults: a little is better than none. *J Hypertens*, August 2020; 38(8):1466–73. Doi: 10.1097/HJH.0000000000002415. PMID: 32102048

10. Pescatello LS, Franklin BA, Fagard R et al. American College of Sports Medicine position stand: Exercise and hypertension. *Med Sci Sports Exerc*, March 2004; 36(3):533–53

11. Joseph G, Marott J, Toorp-Pedersen C et al. Dose-response association between level of physical activity and mortality in normal, elevated and high blood pressure. *Hypertens*, 2019; 74:1307–15

12. Eckel RH, Jakicic JM, Ard JD et al. 2013 AHA/ACC guideline on lifestyle to reduce cardiovascular risk. *J Amer Coll Cardiol*, 2014; 63:25 Part B

13. Pescatello LS. Exercise measures up to medication as hypertensive therapy: its value has long been underestimated. December 2018; bjsports-2018-100359; Doi: 10.1136/bjsports-2018-100359

14. Naci H, Salcher-Konrad M, Dias S et al. How does exercise treatment compare with antihypertensive medications? A network meta-analysis of 391 randomised controlled trials assessing exercise and medication effects on systolic blood pressure. *Br J Sports Med*, 2018; 0:1–2. Doi: 10.1136/bjsports-2018-099921

15. Brook RD, Appel LJ, Rubenfire M et al. Beyond medications and diet: alternative approaches to lowering blood pressure. A scientific statement from the American Heart Association. *Hypertension*, 2013; 61:00–00

16. Dimeo F, Pagonas N, Seibert F et al. Aerobic Exercise Reduces Blood Pressure in Resistant Hypertension. *Hypertension*, 2012; 60:653–58

Dyslipidaemia

1. Park YM, Sui X, Liu J et al. The effect of cardiorespiratory fitness on age related lipids and lipoproteins. *J Amer Coll Cardiol*, 2015; 65:2091–100

2. Kelly GA, Kelley JS, Tran ZV. Walking, lipids, and lipoproteins: a meta-analysis of randomized controlled trials. *Prev Med*, 2004; 38:651–61

3. Leon AS, Sanchez OA. Response of blood lipids to exercise training alone or combined with dietary intervention. *Med Sci Sports Exerc*, 2001; 33:S502–15

4. Varady KA, Jones PJ. Combination Diet and Exercise Interventions for the Treatment of Dyslipidemia: an Effective Preliminary Strategy to Lower Cholesterol Levels? *J Nutrit*, 2005; 135:1829–35

5. Kelley G, Kelley K, Roberts S, Haskell W. Combined Effects of Aerobic Exercise and Diet on Lipids and Lipoproteins in Overweight and Obese Adults: A Meta-Analysis. *J Obesity*, 2012. http://dx.doi.org/10.1155/2012/985902

6. Kokkinos PF, Faselis C, Myers J et al. Interactive effects of fitness and statin treatment on mortality risk in verterans with dyslipidaemia: a cohort study. *Lancet*, 2012; 381:394–9

7. Eckel RH, Jakicic JM, Ard JD et al. 2013 AHA/ACC guideline on lifestyle management to reduce cardiovascular risk. *J Amer Coll Cardiol*, 2014; 63

Diabetes

1. International Diabetes Federation Figures for diabetes in adults aged 20–79, 2013/14

2. www.diabetes.co.uk

3. Espeland M. Reduction in Weight and Cardiovascular Disease Risk Factors in Individuals With Type 2 Diabetes: One-Year Results of the Look AHEAD Trial. *Diabetes Care*, March 2007. https://doi.org/10.2337/dc07-0048

4. Knowler WC, Barrett-Connor E, Fowler SE et al. Reduction in the incidence of type 2 diabetes with lifestyle intervention or metformin. *N Engl J Med*, 7 February 2002; 346(6):393–403

5. Orozco LJ, Buchleitner AM, Gimenez-Perez G et al. Exercise or exercise and diet for preventing type 2 diabetes mellitus. Cochrane Database of Systematic Reviews, 16 July 2008; (3):CD003054. Doi: 10.1002/14651858.CD003054.pub3. Update in: Cochrane Database of Systematic Reviews, 4 December 2017; 12:CD003054. PMID: 18646086

6. Tuomilehto J, Lindström J, Eriksson, JG et al. Prevention of Type 2 Diabetes Mellitus by Changes in Lifestyle among Subjects with Impaired Glucose Tolerance. *N Eng J Med*, 2016; 344:1343–50

7. Mutie P, Drake I, Ericson U et al. Different domains of self-reported physical activity and risk of type 2 diabetes in a population-based Swedish cohort: the Malmö diet and Cancer study. *BMC Public Health*, 20, 261 (2020). https://doi.org/10.1186/s12889-020-8344-2

8. Mielke GI, Bailey TG, Burton NW, Brown WJ. Participation in sports/recreational activities and incidence of hypertension, diabetes, and obesity in adults. *Scand J Med Sci Sports*, December 2020; 30(12):2390–98. Doi: 10.1111/sms.13795. Epub 25 August 2020. PMID: 32757327.

9. Naci H, Salcher-Konrad M, Dias S et al. How does exercise treatment compare with antihypertensive medications? A network meta-analysis of 391 randomised controlled trials assessing exercise and medication effects on systolic blood pressure. *Br J Sports Med*, 2018; 0:1–2. Doi: 10.1136/bjsports-2018-099921

10. Yerramalla MS, Fayosse A, Dugravot A et al. Association of moderate and vigorous physical activity with incidence of type 2 diabetes and subsequent mortality: 27 year follow-up of the Whitehall II study. *Diabetologia*, March 2020; 63(3):537–48. Doi: 10.1007/s00125-019-05050-1

11. Mutie P, Drake I, Ericson U et al. Op. cit.

12. Hemmingsen B, Gimenez-Perez G, Mauricio D et al. Diet, physical activity or both for prevention or delay of type 2 diabetes mellitus and its associated complications in people at increased risk of developing type 2 diabetes. Cochrane Database of Systematic Reviews, 2017. https://doi.org/10.1002/14651858.CD003054.pub4

13. Christian K, Roberts CK, Barnard RJ. Effects of exercise and diet on chronic disease. *Journal of Applied Physiology*, 2005; 98:3–30. Doi: 10.1152/japplphysiol.00852.2004

14. McInnes N, Smith A, Otto R et al. Piloting a remission strategy in Type 2 Diabetes: Results of a randomized controlled trial. *Journal of Clinical Endocrinology & Metabolism*, 2017; 102:1595–605

15. Lean ME, Leslie WS, Barnes AC et al. Primary care-led weight management for remission of type 2 diabetes (DIRECT): an open-label, cluster-randomised trial. *Lancet*, 2017:391:541–51

16. Colberg S, Sigal R, Yardley J et al. Physical Activity/Exercise and Diabetes: A Position Statement of the American Diabetes Association Diabetes Care. November 2016; 39(11) 2065–79. Doi: 10.2337/dc16-1728

17. Barbosa A, Brito J, Figueiredo P et al. Football can tackle type 2 diabetes: a systematic review of the health effects of recreational football practice in individuals with prediabetes and type 2 diabetes. *Res Sports Med*, May–June 2021; 29(3):303-321. Doi: 10.1080/15438627.2020.1777417.

18. Martenstyn J, King M, Rutherford C. Impact of weight loss interventions on patient-reported outcomes in overweight and obese adults with type 2 diabetes: a systematic review. *J Behav Med*, December 2020; 43(6):873–91. Doi: 10.1007/s10865-020-00140-7

19. Pi-Sunyer X. The Look AHEAD Trial: A Review and Discussion of Its Outcomes. *Curr Nutr Rep*, December 2014; 3(4): 387–91

20. Yerramalla MS, Fayosse A, Dugravot A et al. Op. cit.

The metabolic syndrome

1. Grundy SM, Brewer HB, Cleeman JI et al. *Definition of Metabolic Syndrome*. Report of the National Heart, Lung, and Blood Institute/American Heart Association Conference on Scientific Issues Related to Definition Circulation. 2004; 109:433-43 https://www.nhs.uk/conditions/metabolic-syndrome/

2. Galassi A, Reynolds K, He J. Metabolic syndrome and risk of cardiovascular disease: a meta-analysis. *Am J Med*, October 2006; 119(10):812–19

3. Ekelund U, Brage S, Franks PW et al. Physical activity energy expenditure predicts progression toward the metabolic syndrome independently of aerobic fitness in middle-aged healthy Caucasians: the Medical Research Council Ely Study. *Diabetes Care*, 2005; 28:1195–200. Doi:10.2337/diacare.28.5.1195

4. Berentzen T, Petersen L, Pedersen O et al. Long term effects of leisure time physical activity on risk of insulin resistance and impaired glucose tolerance, allowing for body weight history, in Danish men. *Diabet Med*, 2007; 24:63–72

5. Ingle L, Mellis M, Brodie D, Sandercock GR. Associations between cardiorespiratory fitness and the metabolic syndrome in British men. *Heart*. Doi: 10.1136/heartjnl-2016-3101420

6. Hassinen M, Lakka TA, Savonen K et al. Cardiorespiratory fitness as a feature of metabolic syndrome in older men and women. *Diabetes Care*, 2008; 31:1242–7

7. Katzmarzyk PT, Leon AS, Wilmore JH et al. Targeting the metabolic syndrome with exercise: evidence from the HERITAGE family study. *Med Sci Sports Exerc*, 2003; 35:1703–9

8. Johnson JJ, Slentz C, Houmard J et al. Exercise training amount and intensity effects on metabolic syndrome. *Am J Cardiol*, 2007; 100:1759–66

Coronary heart disease (CHD)

1. British Heart Foundation Factsheet, 2015

2. Morris JN, Heady JA, Raffle PA et al. Coronary heart-disease and physical activity of work. *Lancet*, 1953; 265:1111–20

3. Morris J, Clayton D, Everitt M et al. Exercise in leisure time: coronary attack and death rates. *Br Heart J*, 1990; 63:325–34

4. Paffenbarger RS, Hale WE. Work activity and coronary heart mortality. *N Eng J Med*, 1975; 292:545–50

5. Paffenbarger JR, Wing AL, Hyde RT. Physical activity as an index of heart attack risk in college alumni. *Am J Epidemiol*, 1978; 108:161–75

6. Sui X, LaMonte M, Blair S. Cardiorespiratory fitness as a predictor of nonfatal cardiovascular events in asymptomatic women and men. *Am J Epidemiol*, 2007; 165:1413

7. Eckel RH, Jakicic JM, Ard JD et al. 2013 AHA/ACC guideline on lifestyle management to reduce cardiovascular risk, *Circulation*, 2014; 129:S76-s99. https://doi.org/10.1161/01.cir.0000437740.48606.d1

8. Tanasescu M, Leitzmann MF, Rimm EB et al. Exercise type and intensity in relation to coronary heart disease in men. *JAMA*, 23–30 October 2002; 288(16):1994–2000. Doi: 10.1001/jama.288.16.1994. PMID: 12387651

9. Blair SN, Kohl HW, Barlow CE et al. Changes in physical fitness and all-cause mortality. A prospective study of healthy and unhealthy men. *JAMA*, 1995; 273:1093–8

10. Kodama S, Saito K, Tanaka S et al. Cardiorespiratory fitness as a quantitative predictor of all-cause mortality and cardiovascular events in healthy men and women: a meta-analysis. *JAMA*, 20 May 2009; 301(19):2024–35. Doi: 10.1001/jama.2009.681. PMID: 19454641

11. Franco OH, de Laet C, Peeters A et al. Effects of physical activity on life expectancy with cardiovascular disease. *Arc Intern Med*, 2005; 165:2355–60

12. Mozaffarian D, Benjamin E, Go A et al. Heart disease and stroke statistics – 2015 update: a report from the American Heart Association. *Circulation*, 2015; 131:e29–322

13. Lee IM, Shiroma EJ, Lobelo F et al. Effect of physical inactivity on major non-communicable diseases worldwide: an analysis of burden of disease and life expectancy. *Lancet*, 21 July 2012; 380(9838):219–29

14. Zhao M, Veeranki S P, Magnussen C G, Xi B. Recommended physical activity and all cause and cause specific mortality in US adults: prospective cohort study, *BMJ*, 2020; 370:m2031. Doi: 10.1136/bmj.m2031

15. Heberden, W. Some account of a disorder of the breast. *Medical Transactions. The Royal College of Physicians of London*, 1772:2: 59–67

16. Hellerstein HK, Goldston E. Rehabilitation of patients with heart disease. *Post Grad Med*, 1954; 15:265–78

17. Hellerstein HK. Exercise therapy in coronary disease. *Bull NY Academ Med*, 1968; 44:1028–47

18. Taylor RS, Brown A, Ebrahim S et al. Exercise-based rehabilitation for patients with coronary heart disease: systematic review and meta-analysis of randomised controlled trials. *Am J Med*, 2004; 116:682–92

19. Clark AM, Hartling L, Vandermeer B et al. Meta-analysis: secondary prevention programs for patients with coronary disease. *Ann Intern Med*, 2005; 143:659–72

20. Hung RK, Al-Mulla MH, McEvoy JW et al. Prognostic value of exercise capacity in patients with coronary artery disease: the FIT (Henry Ford Exercise Testing) project. *Mayo Clin Proc*, 2014; 12:1644–54

21. Kavanagh T, Mertens TJ, Hamm LF et al. Prediction of long-term prognosis in 12 169 men referred for cardiac rehabilitation. *Circulation*, 2002; 106:666–71

22. Nichols S, Taylor C, Goodman T et al. Routine exercise-based cardiac rehabilitation does not increase aerobic fitness: a care Cr study. *Int J Cardiol*, 2020; 305:25–34. Doi: 10.1016/j.ijcard.2020.01.044

23. Jennings CS, Kotseva K, Bassett P et al. ASPIRE-3-PREVENT Investigators. ASPIRE-3-PREVENT: a cross-sectional survey of preventive care after a coronary event across the UK. *Open Heart*, April 2020; 7(1):e001196. Doi: 10.1136/openhrt-2019-001196 PMID: 32354740; PMCID: PMC7228656

24. Cook R, Davidson P, Martin R. Cardiac rehabilitation for heart failure can improve quality of life and fitness. *BMJ*, 2019; 367:l5456. Doi: 10.1136/bmj.l5456

Peripheral vascular disease

1. Bhuva AN, D'Silva A, Torlasco C et al. Training for a First-Time Marathon Reverses Age-Related Aortic Stiffening. *J Am Coll Cardiol*, 7 January 2020; 75(1):60–71. Doi: 10.1016/j.jacc.2019.10.045. PMID: 31918835

2. Morley RL, Sharma A, Horsch AD et al. Peripheral artery disease. *BMJ*, 2018; 360:j5842

3. Kumagai H, Yoshikawa T, Myoenzono K et al. Role of high physical fitness in deterioration of male sexual function in Japanese adult men. *J Men's Health*, 2019. Doi: org/10.1177/1557988319849171

4. Gardner AW, Poehlman ET. Exercise rehabilitation programmes for the treatment of claudication pain. A meta-analysis. *JAMA* ,1995; 274:975–80

5. Frazzitta G, Maestri R, Bertotti G et al. Intensive rehabilitation treatment in early Parkinson's disease: a randomised pilot study with a 2-year follow up. *Neurorehabil*, 2015; 29:123–31

6. Lane R, Harwood A, Watson L, Leng GC. Exercise for intermittent claudication. Cochrane Database of Systematic Reviews, 2017; Issue 12. CD000990. Doi: 10.1002/14651858.CD000990.pub4

Stroke

1. I-Min L, Hennekens CH, Berger K et al. Exercise and risk of stroke in male physicians. *Stroke*, 1999; 30:1–6

2. Sacco RL, Gan R, Boden-Albala B et al. Leisure time physical activity and ischemic stroke risk. *Stroke*, 1998; 29:380–7

3. Hayes S, Forbes JF, Celis-Morales C et al. Association Between Walking Pace and Stroke Incidence: Findings From the UK Biobank Prospective Cohort Study. *Stroke*, May 2020; 51(5):1388–95. Doi: 10.1161/STROKEAHA.119.028064. Epub 17 April 2020. PMID: 32299326

4. Lee CD, Blair SN. Cardiorespiratory fitness and stroke mortality in men. *Med Sci Sports Excer*, 2002; 34:592–5

5. Pandey A, Patel MR, Willis B et al. *Association between Midlife Cardiorespiratory Fitness and Risk of Stroke*. The Cooper Center Longitudinal Study. Doi: 10.1161/STROKEAHA.115.011532

6. Harris JE, Eng JJ. Strength training improves upper-limb function in individuals with stroke: a meta-analysis. *Stroke*, 2010; 41:136–40

7. Luker J, Lynch E, Bernhardsson S et al. *Stroke Survivors' Experiences of Physical Rehabilitation: A Systematic Review of Qualitative Studies*. September 2015; 96(9):1698–708.e10. Doi: 10.1016/j.apmr.2015.03.017. Epub 3 April 2015. PMID: 25847387.https://doi.org/10.1016/j.apmr.2015.03.017

8. Saunders DH, Greig CA, Mead GE. Physical activity and exercise after stroke. *Stroke*, 2014; 45:3742–47

9. Saunders DH, Sanderson M, Brazzelli M et al. Physical fitness training for stroke patients. Cochrane Database of Systematic Reviews, 2013; 10:CD003316. Doi: 10.1002/14651858.CD003316.pub5

10. Cumming TB, Tyedin K, Churilov L et al. The effect of physical activity on cognitive function after stroke: a systematic review. *Int Psychogeriatr*, 2012; 24:557–67

11. Reed M, Harrington R, Duggan A, Wood VA. Meeting stroke survivors' perceived needs: a qualitative study of a community-based exercise and education scheme. *Clin Rehabil*, 2010; 24:16–25

Parkinson's disease

1. Fang X, Han D, Cheng Q et al. Association of levels of physical activity with risk of Parkinson's disease. A systematic review and meta-analysis. *JAMA* Network open: 1:2018.e182421

2. Müller J, Myers J. Association between physical fitness, cardiovascular risk factors, and Parkinson's disease. *Eur J Prev Cardiol*, September 2018; 25(13):1409–15. Doi: 10.1177/2047487318771168. Epub April 2018. PMID: 29667433

3. Goodwin VA, Richards SH, Taylor RS et al. The effectiveness of exercise interventions for people with Parkinson's disease: a systematic review and meta-analysis. *Mov Disord*, 15 April 2008; 23(5):631–40. Doi: 10.1002/mds.21922. PMID: 18181210

4. Mehrholz J, Kugler J, Storch A et al. Treadmill training for patients with Parkinson's disease. Cochrane Database of Systematic Reviews, 2015; Issue 8. Art. No.: CD007830. Doi: 10.1002/14651858.CD007830.pub3

5. Choi H, Cho K, Jin C et al. Exercise Therapies for Parkinson's Disease: A Systematic Review and Meta-Analysis. *Parkinson's Disease*, Vol. 2020; Article ID 2565320, https://doi.org/10.1155/2020/2565320

6. Schootemeijer S, van der Kolk NM, Bloem BR, de Vries NM. Current Perspectives on Aerobic Exercise in People with Parkinson's Disease. *Neurotherapeutics*, October 2020; 17(4):1418-1433. Doi: 10.1007/s13311-020-00904-8. PMID: 32808252; PMCID: PMC7851311

7. Armstrong M, Okun M. Diagnosis and Treatment of Parkinson Disease. *JAMA*, 2020; 323(6):548–60. Doi: 1: 0.1001/jama.2019.22360

8. Anderson P. Boxing Helps Knock Out Nonmotor Parkinson's Symptoms. ANN Annual meeting. *Medscape Neurology Reviews*, April 2020

9. Sasser L. Picking up a pingpong paddle may benefit people with Parkinson's. American Academy of Neurology, *Science Daily*, 25 February 2020. https://brainandmemoryhealth.com/ping-pong-for-brain-health/

Psychological ill health

1. Ayuso-Mateos JL, Vázquez-Barquero JL, Dowrick C et al. ODIN Group. Depressive disorders in Europe: prevalence figures from the ODIN study. *Br J Psychiatry*, October 2001; 179:308–16. Doi: 10.1192/bjp.179.4.308. PMID: 11581110

2. Goldberg D, Lecrubier Y. Form and frequency of mental disorders across centres. In *Mental Illness in General Health Care: An International Study* (eds N Sartorius, TB Ustun). John Wiley, on behalf of the World Health Organization, 1995

3. Harvey S, Overland S, Hatch S et al. Exercise and the Prevention of Depression: Results of the HUNT Cohort Study. Online 3 Oct 2017. https://doi.org/10.1176/appi.ajp.2017.16111223

4. De Moor MHM, Beem AL, Stubbe JH et al Regular exercise, anxiety, depression and personality: A population-based study. *PrevMed*, 2006; 42:273–79

5. Hassmen P, Koivula N, Uutela A. Physical exercise and psychological well-being: a population study in Finland. *Prev Med*, 2000; 30:17–25

6. Snehal M, Pereira P, Geoffroy M-C, Power C. Depressive symptoms and physical activity during 3 decades in adult life. *JAMA Psychiatry*, 2014; 71:1373–80

7. Mammen G, Faulkner G. Physical Activity and the Prevention of Depression a Systematic Review of Prospective Studies. *Am J Prevent. Med*, 2013; 4:649–57

8. Chekroud SR, Gueorguiva R, Zheutlin AB et al. Association between physical exercise and mental health in 1.2 million individuals in the USA between 2011 and 2015: a cross-sectional study. *Lancet Psychiatry*, 2018; 9:739–46

9. Bennie, J A, De Cocker, K, Biddle, SJH, Teychenne, MJ. Joint and dose-dependent associations between aerobic and muscle-strengthening activity with depression : a cross-sectional study of 1.48 million adults between 2011 and 2017. *Depression and Anxiety*, 2020; 37(2), 166–78. https://doi.org/10.1002/da.22986

10. Pirkis J, Currier D, Carlin J et al. Cohort Profile: Ten to Men (the Australian Longitudinal Study on Male Health). *Int J Epidemiol*, 1 June 2017; 46(3):793–94i. Doi: 10.1093/ije/dyw055. PMID: 27686951

11. Kandola A, Lewis G, Osborn DPJ et al. Depressive symptoms and objectively measured physical activity and sedentary behaviour throughout adolescence: a prospective cohort study. *Lancet Psychiatry*, March 2020; 7(3):262–71. Doi: 10.1016/S2215-0366(20)30034-1

12. Schuch FB, Stubbs B, Meyer J et al. Physical activity protects from incident anxiety: A meta-analysis of prospective cohort studies. *Depress Anxiety*, September 2019; 36(9):846–58. Doi: 10.1002/da.22915

13. Kandola A, Ashdown-Franks G, Stubbs B et al. The association between cardiorespiratory fitness and the incidence of common mental health disorders: A systematic review and meta-analysis. *J Affect Disord*, 1 October 2019; 257:748–57. Doi: 10.1016/j.jad.2019.07.088

14. Cooney GM, Dwan K, Greig CA et al. Exercise for depression. Cochrane Database of Systematic Reviews, 12 September 2013; (9):CD004366. Doi: 10.1002/14651858.CD004366.pub6. PMID: 24026850

15. Carter T, Morres ID, Meade O, Callaghan P. The Effect of Exercise on Depressive Symptoms in Adolescents: A Systematic Review and Meta-Analysis. *J Am Acad Child Adolesc Psychiatry*, July 2016; 55(7):580–90. Doi: 10.1016/j.jaac.2016.04.016

16. Helgadóttir B, Forsell Y, Hallgren M et al. Long-term effects of exercise at different intensity levels on depression: A randomized controlled trial. *Prev Med*, December 2017; 105:37–46. Doi: 10.1016/j.ypmed.2017.08.008

17. Perez-Sousa, MA, Olivares, PR, Gonzalez-Guerrero, JL et al. Effects of an exercise program linked to primary care on depression in elderly: fitness as mediator of the improvement. *Qual Life Res*, 2020; 29, 1239–1246. https://doi.org/10.1007/s11136-019-02406-3

18. Mota-Pereira J, Silverio J, Carvalho S et al. Moderate exercise improves depression parameters in treatment-resistant patients with major depressive disorder. *J Psychiatr Res*, August 2011; 45(8):1005–11. Doi: 10.1016/j.jpsychires.2011.02.005

19. Ströhle A. Physical activity, exercise, depression and anxiety disorders. *J Neural Transm* (Vienna), June 2009; 116(6):777–84. Doi: 10.1007/s00702-008-0092-x

20. Hallgren M, Helgadóttir B, Herring MP et al. Exercise and internet-based cognitive-behavioural therapy for depression: multicentre randomised controlled trial with 12-month follow-up. *Br J Psychiatry*, November 2016; 209(5):414–20. Doi: 10.1192/bjp.bp.115.177576

21. Royal College of Psychiatrists. http://www.rcpsych.ac.uk/healthadvice/treatmentswellbeing/physicalactivity.aspx

22. Parkinson J. Review of scales of positive mental health validated for use with adults in the UK. NHSHealthScotland, 2008

23. Halliday, A et al. Can physical activity help explain the gender gap in adolescent mental health? A cross-sectional exploration. *Mental Health and Physical Activity*, 2 February 2019; 8–18. Doi.org/10.1016/j.mhpa.2019.02.002

24. Kim, YS, Park, YS, Allegrante, J et al. Relationship between physical activity and general mental health. *Prev Med*, 2012; 55(5), 458–63. Doi: https://doi.org/10.1016/j.ypmed.2012.08.021

25. Qu X. Empirical analysis of the influence of physical exercise on psychological stress of college students. *Revista Argentina de Clínica Psicológica*, 2020. Doi: 10.24205/03276716.2020., Vol. XXIX, N°2, 1443-1451386

26. Fluetsch N, Levy C, Tallon L. The relationship of physical activity to mental health: A 2015 behavioral risk factor surveillance system data analysis. *J Affect Disord*, 15 June 2019; 253:96–101. Doi: 10.1016/j.jad.2019.04.086

27. Tamminena N, Jaakko Reinikainenb J, Appelqvist-Schmidlechner K et al. Associations of physical activity with positive mental health: A population based study. *Mental Health and Physical Activity*, Volume 18, March 2020; 100319

Dementia

1. Alty J, Farrow M, Lawler K et al. Exercise and dementia prevention. Doi: 10.1136/practneurol-2019-002335

2. Alzheimer's Research UK, 2017

3. Andel R, Crowe M, Pedersen NL et al. Physical Exercise at Midlife and Risk of Dementia Three Decades Later: A Population-Based Study of Swedish Twins. *Journal of Gerontology*, 2008; Vol. 63A, No. 1, 62–6

4. Hamer M, Chida Y. Physical activity and risk of cognitive decline. *Psychol Med*, 2009; 39:3–11

5. Defina LF, Willis BL, Radford NB et al. The association between midlife cardiorespiratory fitness levels and later-life dementia: a cohort study. *Ann Intern Med*, 2013; 158:162–8

6. Hörder H, Johansson L, Guo X et al. Midlife cardiovascular fitness and dementia. *Neurology*, 2018; 10.1212/WNL.0000000000005290

7. Damiel L et al. www.isrctn.com/ISRTCN89898870

8. Elwood P, Galante J , Pickering J et al. Healthy Lifestyles Reduce the Incidence of Chronic Diseases and Dementia: Evidence from the Caerphilly Cohort Study PloS One, 2013; journals.plos.org

9. Northey JM, Cherbuin N, Pumpa K et al. Exercise interventions for cognitive function in adults older than 50: a systematic review with meta-analysis. *Brit J Sports Med*, 2017; Doi: 10.1136/bjsports-2016-096587

10. Kivimaki M, Singh-Menoux A, Pentti J et al. Physical inactivity, cardiometabolic disease, and risk of dementia: an individual-participant meta-analysis. *BMJ*, 2019; 365:l1495

11. Erickson KI, Weinstein AM, Lopez OL. Physical activity, brain plasticity, and Alzheimer's disease. *Archives of Medical Research*, 2012; 43(8):615–21

12. Thomas AG, Dennis A, Bandettine PA et al. The Effects of Aerobic Activity on Brain Structure. *Front Psychol*, 2012; 3:86

13. Ahlskog JE, Geda YE, Graff-Radford NR, Petersen RC. Physical exercise as a preventive or disease-modifying treatment of dementia and brain aging. *Mayo Clin Proc*, September 2011; 86(9):876–84. Doi: 10.4065/mcp.2011.0252. PMID: 21878600; PMCID: PMC3258000

14. Andrews SC, Curtin D, Hawi Z et al. Intensity Matters: High-intensity Interval Exercise Enhances Motor Cortex Plasticity More Than Moderate Exercise. *Cereb Cortex*, 10 January 2020; 30(1):101–12. Doi: 10.1093/cercor/bhz075. PMID: 31041988

15. Erikson S, Voss MW, Prakash RS et al. Exercise training increases size of hippocampus and improves memory. *PNAS*, 2011; 108:3017–22

16. Forbes D, Forbes SC, Blake CM et al. Exercise programs for people with dementia. Cochrane Database of Systematic Reviews, 2015

17. Gomes-Osman J, Cabral DF, Morris T et al. Exercise for cognitive brain health in aging. A systematic review for an evaluation of dose. *Neurology*, 2018; 9:257–65

18. Zheng G, Xia R, Zhou W et al. Aerobic exercise ameliorates cognitive function in older adults with mild cognitive impairment: a systematic review and meta-analysis of randomised controlled trials. *British Journal of Sports Medicine*, 2016; 50:1443–50

19. Biazus-Sehn LF, Schuch FB, Firth J, Stigger FS. Effects of physical exercise on cognitive function of older adults with mild cognitive impairment: A systematic review and meta-analysis. *Arch Gerontol Geriatr*, July–August 2020; 89:104048. Doi: 10.1016/j.archger.2020.104048

20. Lam FM, Huang MZ, Liao LR et al.Physical exercise improves strength, balance, mobility, and endurance in people with cognitive impairment and dementia: a systematic review. *J Physiother*, January 2018; 64(1):4–15. Doi: 10.1016/j.jphys.2017.12.001

21. Sampaio, A, Marques-Aleixo, I, Seabra, A et al. Physical fitness in institutionalized older adults with dementia: association with cognition, functional capacity and quality of life. *Aging Clin Exp Res*, 2020; 32, 2329–38. https://doi.org/10.1007/s40520-019-01445-7

22. Machado FB, Silva N, Farinatti P et al. Effectiveness of Multicomponent Exercise Interventions in Older Adults with Dementia: A Meta-Analysis. *Gerontologist*, 11 July 2020; gnaa091. Doi: 10.1093/geront/gnaa091

Lung disease

1. Rochester CL, Holland AE. Pulmonary Rehabilitation and Improved Survival for Patients with COPD. *JAMA*, 12 May 2020; 323(18):1783–5. Doi: 10.1001/jama.2020.4436. PMID: 32396172

2. McCarthy B, Casey D, Devane D et al. Pulmonary rehabilitation for chronic obstructive pulmonary disease. Cochrane Database of Systematic Reviews, 23 February 2015; (2):CD003793. Doi: 10.1002/14651858.CD003793.pub3. PMID: 25705944

3. Rochester CL, Holland AE. Op. cit.

4. Bolton CE, Bevan-Smith EF, Blakey JD et al. British Thoracic Society Pulmonary Rehabilitation Guideline Development Group; British Thoracic Society Standards of Care Committee. British Thoracic Society guideline on pulmonary rehabilitation in adults. *Thorax*, September 2013; 68 Suppl 2:ii1–30. Doi: 10.1136/thoraxjnl-2013-203808

5. Jaakkola MS, Aalto SAM, Hyrkäs-Palmu H, Jaakkola JJK. Association between regular exercise and asthma control among adults: The population-based Northern Finnish Asthma Study. *PLoS One*, 23 January 2020; 15(1):e0227983

6. Nici L, Donner C , Wouters E et al. American Thoracic Society/European Respiratory Society Statement on Pulmonary Rehabilitation. *American Journal of Respiratory and Critical Care Medicine*, 2005; 173, Issue 12https://doi.org/10.1164/rccm.200508-1211ST

7. Geidl, W, Schlesinger, S, Mino, E et al. Dose–response relationship between physical activity and mortality in adults with noncommunicable diseases: a systematic review and meta-analysis of prospective observational studies. *Int J Behav Nutr Phys Act*, 17, 109, 2020. https://doi.org/10.1186/s12966-020-01007-5

Cancer

1. World Cancer Research Fund (WCRF) Panel. *Food, Nutrition, Physical Activity, and the Prevention of Cancer: A Global Perspective*. World Cancer Research Fund, 2007

2. Lee IM. Physical activity and cancer prevention – data from epidemiologic studies. *Med Sci Sports Exerc*, November 2003; 35(11):1823–7. Doi: 10.1249/01.MSS.0000093620.27893.23. PMID: 14600545

3. Voskuil DW, Monninkhof EM, Elias SG et al. Task force physical activity and cancer. Physical activity and endometrial cancer risk, a systematic review of current evidence. *Cancer Epidemiol Biomarkers Prev*, 2007; 16:639–48

4. Parkin D. Cancers attributable to inadequate physical exercise in the UK in 2010. *Br J Cancer*, 6 December 2011; 105 (Suppl 2–): S38S41

5. Moore SC, Lee I-M, Weiderpass E et al. Association of leisure-time physical activity with risk of 26 types of cancer in 1.44 million adults. *JAMA Intern Med*, 2016; 176:816–25

6. World Cancer Research Fund Annual Review, 2009–10

7. Vainshelboim B, Lima RM, Myers J. Cardiorespiratory fitness and cancer in women: A prospective pilot study. *J Sport Health Sci*, 2019; 8(5):457–62. Doi:10.1016/j.jshs.2019.02.001

8. Sui X, Lee DC, Matthews CE et al. Influence of cardiorespiratory fitness on lung cancer mortality. *Med Sci Sports Exerc*, 2010; 42(5):872–8. Doi:10.1249/MSS.0b013e3181c47b65

9. Zhao M, Veeranki S, Costan G et al. Recommended physical activity and all cause and cause specific mortality in US adults: prospective cohort study. *BMJ*, 2020; 370:m2031. http://dx.doi.org/10.1136/bmj.m2031

10. Kyrgiou M, Kalliala I, Markozannes G et al. Adiposity and cancer at major anatomical sites. *BMJ*, 2017; 356:j477

11. Lauby-Secretan B, Scoccianti C, Loomis D et al. Body fatness and cancer – viewpoint of the IARC working group. *N Engl J Med*, 2016; 375:794–8. Doi: 10.1056/NEJMsr1606602

12. Teras LR, Patel AV, Wang M et al. Sustained Weight Loss and Risk of Breast Cancer in Women 50 Years and Older: A Pooled Analysis of Prospective Data. *J Natl Cancer Inst*, 1 September 2020; 112(9):929–37. Doi: 10.1093/jnci/djz226. PMID: 31845728; PMCID: PMC7492760

13. Himbert C, Klossner N, Coletta A et al. Exercise and lung cancer surgery: A systematic review of randomized-controlled trials. *Critical Reviews in Oncology/Hematology*, Vol. 156, December 2020; 103086. https://doi.org/10.1016/j.critrevonc.2020.103086

14. Hayes SC, Steele M, Spence R et al. 2017. Can exercise influence survival following breast cancer: Results from a randomised, controlled trial. *Journal of Clinical Oncology*, 2017; 35:15_suppl, 10067–10067

15. McNeely ML, Campbell KL, Rowe BH et al. Effects of exercise on breast cancer patients and survivors: a systematic review and meta-analysis. *CMAJ*, 2006; 175:34–41

16. Segal R, Zwaal C, Green E et al. Exercise for people with cancer: a systematic review. *Curr Oncol*, 2017; 24:e290–315

17. Mishra SI, Scherer RW, Snyder C et al. Exercise interventions on health-related quality of life for people with cancer during active treatment. Cochrane Database of Systematic Reviews, 2012

Osteoporosis

1. National Osteoporosis Society. The Osteoporosis Agenda England, 2015

2. Warburton DE, Glendhill N, Quinney A. The effects of changes in musculoskeletal fitness on health. *Can J Appl Physiol*, April 2001; 26(2):161–216. Doi: 10.1139/h01-012. PMID: 11312416

3. Elhakeem A, Heron J, Tobias JH, Lawlor DA. Physical Activity Throughout Adolescence and Peak Hip Strength in Young Adults. *JAMA Netw Open*, 2020; 3(8):e2013463. Doi:10.1001/jamanetworkopen.2020.13463

4. Kujala UM, Kaprio J, Kannus P et al. Physical activity and osteoporotic hip fracture risk in men. *Arch Intern Med*, 2000; 160: 705–8

5. Paganini-Hill A, Chao A, Ross RK, Henderson BE. Exercise and other factors in the prevention of hip fracture: the Leisure World study. *Epidemiology*, January 1991; 2(1):16–25

6. Marks R. Hip fracture epidemiological trends, outcomes, and risk factors, 1970–2009. *Int J Med*, 2010; 3:1–17

7. Haapasalo H, Kannus P, Sievanen H et al. Long-term unilateral loading and bone mineral density and content in female squash players. *Calcif Tissue Int*, 1994; 54:249–55

8. Howe TE, Shea B, Dawson LJ et al. Exercise for preventing and treating osteoporosis in postmenopausal women. *Cochrane Library*, 2011

9. A. Gómez-Cabello A, Ara I, González-Agüero A et al. Effects of Training on Bone Mass in Older Adults. *Sports Med*, 2012; 42: 301–25

Chapter 11 Frailty

1. Fried LP, Tangen CM, Walston J et al. Frailty in older adults: evidence for a phenotype. *J Gerontol A Biol Sci Med Sci*, 2001; 56(3):M146–M156

2. Srithumsuk, W, Kabayama, M, Godai, K et al. Association between physical function and long-term care in community-dwelling older and oldest people: the SONIC study. *Environ Health Prev Med*, 25, 46, 2020. https://doi.org/10.1186/s12199-020-00884-3

3. Doherty TJ. Invited review: Aging and sarcopenia. *J Appl Physiol*, 1985; October 2003; 95(4):1717–27. Doi: 10.1152/japplphysiol.00347.2003. PMID: 12970377

4. English K, Paddon-Jones D. Protecting muscle mass and function in older adults during bed rest. *Curr Opin Clin Nutr Metab Care*, 2010; 13:34–9. Doi: 10.1097/MCO.0b013e328333aa66

5. Fleg JL, Morrell CH, Bos AG et al. Accelerated longitudinal decline of aerobic capacity in healthy older adults. *Circulation*, 2005; 112:674–82

6. Fentem PH, Collins MF, Tuxworth W et al. Allied Dunbar National Fitness Survey. Technical Report. London: Sports Council, 1994

7. Shephard RJ. Maximal oxygen intake and independence in old age. *Br J Sports Med*, 2009; 43:342–6

8. Tidy C, Knott K. Prevention of falls in the elderly. https://patient.info/doctor/prevention-of-falls-in-the-elderly-pro

9. Lazarus NR, Lord JM, Harridge SDR. The relationships and interactions between age, exercise and physiological function. *J Physiol*, 2018. Doi: 10.1113/JP277071

10. English K, Paddon-Jones D. Op. cit.

11. Martínez-Velilla N, Casas-Herrero A, Zambom-Ferraresi F et al. Effect of Exercise Intervention on Functional Decline in Very Elderly Patients During Acute Hospitalization: . A Randomized Clinical Trial. *JAMA Intern Med*, 2019; 179(1):28–36. Doi:10.1001/jamainternmed.2018.4869

12. *Health & Life Expectancies*. Office of National Statistics, 2014

13. Blaha MJ, Hung RK, Dardari Z et al. Age-dependent prognostic value of exercise capacity and derivation of fitness-associated biologic age. *Heart*, March 2016; 102(6):431–7. Doi: 10.1136/heartjnl-2015-308537. Epub 2016 Jan 5. PMID: 26732181

14. Pollock RD, Carter S, Velloso CP et al. An investigation into the relationship between age and physiological function in highly active older adults. *J Physiol*, 1 February 2015; 593(3):657–80; discussion 680. Doi: 10.1113/jphysiol.2014.282863. Epub 6 January 2015. PMID: 25565071; PMCID: PMC4324712

15. Fries JF. Physical activity, the compression of morbidity, and the health of the elderly. *J R Soc Med*, February 1996; 89(2): 64–8

16. Chakravarty EF, Hubert HB, Lingala VB, Fries JF. Reduced disability and mortality among aging runners: a 21-year longitudinal study. *Arch Intern Med*, 2008: 168; 1638–46

17. Singh MA. Exercise comes of age: rationale and recommendations for a geriatric exercise prescription. *J. Gerontol. A Biol. Sci. Med. Sci*, 2002; 57: M262–M282

18. Young A, Dinan S. ABC of sports and exercise medicine. Activity in later life. *Brit Med J*, 2005; 330:189–91

19. Simoes EJ, Kobau R, Kapp J et al. Associations of physical activity and body mass index with activities of daily living in older adults. *J Comm Health*, 2006; 31:45–67

20. Gil-Salcedo A, Dugravot A, Fayosse A et al. Healthy behaviors at age 50 years and frailty at older ages in a 20-year follow-up of the UK Whitehall II cohort: A longitudinal study. *PLoS Med*, 2020; 17(7):e1003147. https://doi.org/10.1371/journal. pmed.1003147

21.Gu MO, Conn VS. Meta-analysis of the effects of exercise interventions on functional status in older adults. *Res in Nursing and Health*, 2008; 31:594–603

22. Theou O, Stathokostas L, Roland KP et al. The effectiveness of exercise interventions for the management of frailty: a systematic review. *J Aging Res*, 4 April 2011; 2011:569194. Doi: 10.4061/2011/569194

23. Pahor M, Guralnik JM, Ambrosius WT et al. Effect of structured physical activity on prevention of major mobility disability in older adults: the LIFE Study Randomized Clinical Trial. *JAMA*, 2014; 311:2387–96

24. Faber M, Bosscher R, Chin A et al. Effects of exercise programs on falls and mobility in frail and prefrail older adults: a multicenter randomized controlled trial. *Arch Phys Med Rehabil*, 2006; 87: 885–96

25. Kojima G, Kendrick D, Skelton DA et al. Frailty predicts short-term incidence of future falls among British community-dwelling older people: a prospective cohort study nested within a randomised controlled trial. *BMC Geriatr*, 2015; 15:155. Doi: 10.1186/s12877-015-0152-7

26. de Vries OJ, Peeters GM, Lips P, Deeg DJ. Does frailty predict increased risk of falls and fractures? A prospective population-based study. *Osteoporos Int*, September 2013; 24(9):2397–403. Doi: 10.1007/s00198-013-2303-z. Epub 22 February 2013. PMID: 23430104

27. El-Khoury F, Cassou B, Charles M-A et al. The effect of fall prevention exercise programmes on fall induced injuries in community dwelling older adults: systematic review and meta-analysis of randomised controlled trials. *BMJ*, 2013; 347:f6234

28. Sherrington C, Fairhall N, Wallbank G et al. Exercise for preventing falls in older people living in the community. Cochrane Database of Systematic Reviews, 2019.
https://doi.org/10.1002/14651858.CD012424.pub2

Chapter 12: Longevity

1. *Health & Life Expectancies.* Office of National Statistics 2014

2. Public Health England, 2017

3. Institute and Faculty of Actuaries, 2018

4. Stofan JR, DiPietro L, Davis D et al. Physical activity patterns associated with cardiorespiratory fitness and reduced mortality: The Aerobics Centre Longitudinal Study. *Am J Public Health*, 2008; 88:1807–13

5. Morris J, Heady J, Raffle P et al. Coronary heart disease and physical activity of work. *Lancet*, 1953; 2:1053

6. Morris J, Clayton D, Everitt M et al. Exercise in leisure time: coronary attack and death rates. *Brit Heart J*, 1990; 63:325–34

7. Franco OH, de Laet C, Peeters A et al. Effects of physical activity on life expectancy with cardiovascular disease. *Arc Intern Med*; 2005; 165:2355–60

8. Clarke PM, Walter SJ, Hayen A et al. Survival of the fittest: retrospective cohort study of the longevity of Olympic medallists in the modern era. *BMJ*, 13 December 2012; 345:e8308. Doi: 10.1136/bmj.e8308

9. Bauman AE, Blair SN. Elite athletes' survival advantage. *BMJ*, 2012; 345:e8338

10. Chakravarty EF, Hubert HB, Lingala VB, Fries JF. Reduced disability and mortality among aging runners: a 21-year longitudinal study. *Arch Intern Med*, 2008; 168:1638–46

11. Lee D, Brellenthin A, Thompson PD et al. Running as a key lifestyle medicine for longevity. *Prog Cardiovasc Dis*, 30 March 2017; pii: S0033–0620(17)30048-8. Doi: 10.1016/j.pcad.2017.03.005

12. Schnohr P, O'Keefe JH, Marott JL et al. Dose of jogging and long-term mortality: the Copenhagen City Heart Study. *J Am Coll Cardiol*, 10 February 2015; 65(5):411-9. Doi: 10.1016/j.jacc.2014.11.023. PMID: 25660917

13. Samitz G, Egger M, Zwahlen M. Domains of physical activity and all-cause mortality: systematic review and dose–response meta-analysis of cohort studies. *Int J Epidemiol*, 2011; 40 (5): 1382–400

14. Lear SA, Hu W, Rangarajan S et al. The effect of physical activity on mortality and cardiovascular disease in 130 000 people from 17 high-income, middle-income, and low-income countries: the PURE study. *Lancet*, 2017; 390:2643–54

15. Moore S, Patel A, Matthews C et al. Leisure Time Physical Activity of Moderate to Vigorous Intensity and Mortality: A Large Pooled Cohort Analysis. *PLOS*, 6 November 2012. Doi.org/10.1371/journal.pmed.1001335

16. Zhao M, Veeranki S, Magnussen C, Bo Xi. Recommended physical activity and all cause and cause specific mortality in US adults: prospective cohort study. *BMJ*, 2020; 370:m2031

17. Chase N, Xuemei S, Blair S. Swimming and All-Cause Mortality Risk Compared With Running, Walking, and Sedentary Habits in Men International. *Journal of Aquatic Research and Education*, 2008; Vol. 2: No. 3, Article 3

18. Celis-Morales CA, Lyall DM, Welsh P et al. Association between active commuting and incident cardiovascular disease, cancer and mortality. *BMJ*, 2017; 357:1456

19. Byberg L, Melhus H, Gedeborg R et al. Total mortality after changes in leisure time physical activity in 50 year old men: 35 year follow-up of population based cohort. *BMJ*, 2009; 338:936

20. Saint-Morris P, Coughlan D, Kelly SP et al. Association of leisure time physical activity across the adult life course with all-cause and cause-specific mortality. *JAMA Netw Open*, 2019; . 2019;2(3):e190355. Doi:10.1001/jamanetworkopen.2019.0355

21. Mok A, Khaw K, Luben R et al. Physical activity trajectories and mortality: population based cohort study. *BMJ*, 2019; 365:l2323. Doi: 10.1136/bmj.l2323

22. Marques A, Gouveira E, Peralta M et al. Cardiorespiratory fitness and telomere length: a systematic review. *Journal of Sports Sciences*, 2020; 38:14, 1690–97. Doi: 10.1080/02640414.2020.1754739

23. Tucker LA. Physical activity and telomere length in U.S. men and women: An NHANES investigation. *Prev Med*, July 2017; 100:145–51. Doi: 10.1016/j.ypmed.2017.04.027. Epub 2017 Apr 24. PMID: 28450121

24. Blair SN. Physical inactivity: the biggest public health problem of the 21st Century. *B J Sports Med*, 2009; 43:1–2

25. Sandvik L, Erikssen J, Thaulow E et al. Physical Fitness as a Predictor of Mortality Among Healthy, Middle-Aged Norwegian Men. *New Eng J Med*, 1993; 328:533–7

26. Kodama S, Saito K, Tanaka S et al. Cardiorespiratory fitness as a quantitative predictor of all-cause mortality and cardiovascular events in healthy men and women: a meta-analysis. *JAMA*, 2009; 3012024–35

27. Blaha MJ, Hung RK, Dardarl Z et al. Age-dependent value of exercise capacity and derivation of fitness associated biologic age. *Heart*, 2016; 102:431–7

28. Mandsanger K, Harb S, Cremer P et al. Association of cardiorespiratory fitness with long-term mortality among adults undergoing exercise treadmill testing. *JAMA*, 2018. Doi: 10.1001/jamanetworkopen.2018.3605

29. Clausen JSR, Marott JL, Holtermann A et al. Midlife Cardiorespiratory Fitness and the Long-Term Risk of Mortality: 46 Years of Follow-Up. *J Am Coll Cardiol*, 28 August 2018; 72(9):987–95. Doi: 10.1016/j.jacc.2018.06.045. PMID: 30139444

30. Kokkinos P, Myers J, Faselis C et al. Exercise capacity and mortality in older men: a 20-year follow-up study. *Circulation*, 2010; 122:790–97

31. Cooper R, Kuh D, Hardy R et al. Objectively measured physical capability levels and mortality: systematic review and meta-analysis. *BMJ*, 2010; 341:c4467

32. Ruiz JR, Sui X, Lobelo F et al. Association between muscular strength and mortality in men: prospective cohort study. *BMJ*, 2008; 337:a439

Chapter 13: The Social and Economic Cost of Sloth

1. O'Keefe JH, Lavie CJ. Run for your life . . . at a comfortable speed and not too far. *Heart*, 2013; 99:516–19

2. Heron L, O'Neill C, McAneney H, et al. Direct healthcare costs of sedentary behaviour in the UK. *J Epidemiol Community Health*, 2019; 73:**625**–9

3. Allender S, Foster C, Scarborough P, and Rayner M. The burden of physical activity related ill health in the UK. *J Epidemiol Community Health*, April 2007; 61(4): 344–8

4. British Heart Foundation. Economic costs of physical inactivity. 2017; bhfactive.org.uk

5. Centre for Economic and Business Research. The economic costs of inactivity in Europe, June 2015. https://cebr.com/reports/the-costs-of-inactivity-in-europe/2015

Chapter 14: Encouraging Exercise

1. Hillsdon M, Foster C, Cavill N et al, for the Health Development Agency. The effectiveness of public health interventions for increasing physical activity among adults: a review of reviews: Evidence briefing, 2nd edn, London: Health Development Agency, 2005

2. Corder K, Sharp S, Jong S et al. Effectiveness and cost-effectiveness of the GoActive intervention to increase physical activity among UK adolescents: A cluster randomised controlled trial. *PLOS*, July 2020. https://doi.org/10.1371/journal.pmed.1003210

3. Kraschnewski JL, Sciamanna CN, Stuckey HL et al. A silent response to the obesity epidemic: Decline in US physician weight counselling. *Med Care*, 2013; 51:186–92

4. Lawlor, Hanratty B. The effectiveness of physical activity advice given in routine primary care consultations: a systematic review. *J Publ Health Med*, 2001; 23:219–26

5. Orrow G, Kinmonth A-L, Sanderson S, Sutton S. Effectiveness of physical activity promotion based in primary care: systematic review and meta-analysis of randomised controlled trials. *BMJ*, 2012; 344:16

6. Craig A, Dinan S, Smith A et al. *NHS: exercise referrals systems: a national quality assurance framework*. Department of Health, 2000

7. Hillsdon M, Foster C, Thorogood M. Interventions for promoting physical activity. Cochrane Database of Systematic Reviews, 2005;(!):CD003180

8. Pavey T, Taylor A, Fox K et al. Effect of exercise referral schemes in primary care on physical activity and improving health outcomes: systematic review and meta-analysis 2011. *BMJ*, 2011; 343:d6462

9. Wade M, Mann S, Copeland RJ, Steele J. Effect of exercise referral schemes upon health and well-being: initial observational insights using individual patient data meta-analysis from the National Referral Database. *J Epidemiol Community Health*, January 2020; 74(1):32–41. Doi: 10.1136/jech-2019-212674. Epub 2019 Nov 18. PMID: 31740446

10. Williams N, Hendry M, France B et al. Effectiveness of exercise-referral schemes to promote physical activity in adults: systematic review. *Brit J Gen Pract*, 2007; 57:979–86

11. Elley CR, Garrett S, Rose SB et al. Cost-effectiveness of exercise on prescription with telephone support among women in general practice over 2 years. *Br J Sports Med*, December 2011; 45(15):1223–9. Doi: 10.1136/bjsm.2010.072439. Epub 16 November 2010. PMID: 21081641

12. Sayburn A. Is lifestyle medicine emerging as a new medical specialty? *BMJ*, 2018; 363:138–9

13. Lawton B, Rose S, Elley C et al. Exercise on prescription for women aged 40–74 recruited through primary care: two year randomised controlled trial. *Brit Med J*, 2008; 337:a2509

14. British Heart Foundation. *Physical activity statistics*, 2015

15. Alberta Center for Active Living. Increasing physical activity and decreasing sedentary behaviour in the workplace. 2015. https://sites.ualberta.ca/~active/workplace/

16. Song Z, Baicker K. Effect of a Workplace Wellness Program on Employee Health and Economic Outcomes: A Randomized Clinical Trial. *JAMA*, 16 April 2019; 321(15):1491–501. Doi: 10.1001/jama.2019.3307. Erratum in: *JAMA*, 17 2019. PMID: 30990549; PMCID: PMC6484807

17. Fazli GS, Moineddin R, Chu A, et al. Neighborhood walkability and pre-diabetes incidence in a multiethnic population. *BMJ Open Diabetes Research & Care*, 2020; 8:e000908. Doi: 10.1136/bmjdrc-2019-000908

18. Aldred R, Goodman A. Low Traffic Neighbourhoods, Car Use, and Active Travel: Evidence from the People and Places Survey of Outer

London Active Travel Interventions. *Transport Findings*, September 2020. https://doi.org/10.32866/001c.17128

19. Active Living Research. https://www.activelivingresearch.org/

20. Sallis JF, Cerin E, Conway TL et al. Physical activity in relation to urban environment in 14 cities worldwide: a cross-sectional study. *Lancet*, 2016. Doi://10.1016/SO140-6736(15)01284-2

21. Gordon-Larsen P, Boone-Heinonen P, Sidney S et al. Active commuting and cardiovascular disease risk. *Arch Intern Med*, 2009; 169:1216–23

22. Celis-Morales CA, Lyall DM, Welsh P et al. Association between active commuting and incident cardiovascular disease, cancer and mortality. *BMJ*, 2017; 357:140

23. Hochsmann C, Muller O, Ambuhl M et al. Novel Smartphone Game Improves Physical Activity Behavior in Type 2 Diabetes. *Am J PrevMed*, July 2019; Vol. 57 (No. 1), 41–50

24. Jakicic JM, Davis KK, Rogers RJ et al. Effect of Wearable Technology Combined With a Lifestyle Intervention on Long-term Weight Loss. The IDEA Randomized Clinical Trial*JAMA*, 2016; 316(11):1161–71. Doi: 10.1001/jama.2016.12858

25. Cramer S. Label food with equivalent exercise to counter obesity. *BMJ*, 2016; 353:i1856

26. Sparling PB, Howard BJ, Dunstan DW, Owen N. Recommendations for physical activity in older adults. *BMJ*, 2015; 350:19–20

27. National Institute for Health Research. *Moving matters – interventions to increase physical activity*. July 2019. Doi: 10.3310/themedreview-03898

28. Hillsdon M, Thorogood M. A systematic review of physical activity promotion strategies. *B J Sports Med*, 1996; 30:84–9

29. McCartney M. Futile exercise. *BMJ*, 2015; 351:23

Chapter 15: Sedentary Behaviour

1. Katzmarzyk P, Powell K, Jakicic J et al. Sedentary Behavior and Health: Update from the 2018 Physical Activity Guidelines Advisory Committee, American College of Sports Med. *Med Sci Sport Exerc*, 2019; 51:1227. Doi: 10.1249/MSS.0000000000001935

2. Owen N. Sedentary behavior: Understanding and influencing adults' prolonged sitting time. *Prev Med*, 2012; 55:535–9

3. Healy GN, Dunstan DW, Salmon J et al. Television time and continuous metabolic risk in physically active adults. *Med Sci Sports Exerc*, 2008; 40:639–45

4. Ussery E, Fulton J, Galuska D. Joint prevalence of sitting time and leisure-time physical activity among US adults, 2015–2016. *JAMA*, 2018; 320:2036–8. Doi: 10.1001/jama.2018.17797

5. Yoo J, Cho J, Baek K et al. Relationship between Smartphone Use Time, Sitting Time, and Fitness Level in University. *Students Exerc Sci*, 2020; 29(2):170–77.. Doi: org/10.15857/ksep.2020.29.2.170

6. Barkley J, Lepp A, Glickman E et al. The Acute Effects of the COVID-19 Pandemic on Physical Activity and Sedentary Behavior in University Students and Employees. *International Journal of Exercise Science*, 2020; 13 (5): 1326–39

7. Gine-Garriga M, Sansano-Nadal, O, Tully, MA et al. Accelerometer-measured sedentary and physical activity time and their correlates in European older adults: the SITLESS study. *The Journals of Gerontology*, Series A, *Biological Sciences and Medical Sciences*, 2020; 75(9), 1754–62. Doi: 10.1093/gerona/glaa016

8. Prince S, Elliott C, Scott K et al. Device-measured physical activity, sedentary behaviour and cardiometabolic health and fitness across occupational groups: a systematic review and meta-analysis. *Int J Behav Nutrit Phys Activity*, 2019. https://doi.org/10.1186/s12966-019-0790-9

9. Diaz KM, Howard VJ, Hutto B et al. Patterns of Sedentary Behavior and Mortality in U.S. Middle-Aged and Older Adults: A National Cohort Study. *Annals Intern Med*, 2017; 167:465–75

10. Ekelund U, Steene-Johannessen J, Brown WJ et al. Does physical activity attenuate, or even eliminate, the detrimental association of sitting time with mortality? A harmonised meta-analysis of data from more than 1 million men and women. *Lancet*, 2016; 388:1302–10

11. Oggioni C, Lara J, Wells J et al. Shifts in population dietary patterns and physical inactivity as determinants of global trends in the prevalence of diabetes: an ecological analysis. *Nutr Metab Cardiovasc Dis*, 2014; 24:1105–11

12. Kulinski J, Kozlitina J, Berry J et al. Sedentary behavior is associated with coronary artery calcification in the Dallas Heart Study. *Journal of the American College of Cardiology*, 2015; 65 (10): A1446. Doi: 10.1016/S0735-1097(15)61446-2

13. Patterson F, Mitchell JA, Dominick G et al. Does meeting physical activity recommendations ameliorate association between television viewing with cardiovascular disease risk? A cross-sectional, population-based analysis. *BMJ Open*, 2020; 10:e036507. Doi: 10.1

14. Biswas A, Oh P, Faulkner G et al. Sedentary time and its association with risk for disease incidence, mortality, and hospitalisation in adults: a systematic review and meta-analysis. *Arch Int Med*, 2015; 162:123–32

15. Gilchrist SC, Howard VJ, Akinyemiju T et al. Association of Sedentary Behavior with Cancer Mortality in Middle-aged and Older US Adults. *JAMA Oncol*, 1 August 2020; 6(8):1210–17. Doi: 10.1001/jamaoncol.2020.2045. PMID: 32556069; PMCID: PMC7303924

16. Heron L, O'Neill C, McAneney H et al. Direct healthcare costs of sedentary behaviour in the UK. *J Epidem Comm Health*. http://dx.doi.org/10.1136/jech-2018-211758

17. Hagger-Johnson G, Gow AJ, Burley V et al. Sitting Time, Fidgeting, and All-Cause Mortality in the UK Women's Cohort Study. *Am J Prev Med*, February 2016; 50(2):154–60. Doi: 10.1016/j.amepre.2015.06.025. Epub 2015 Sep 23. PMID: 26416340

18. Edwardson CL, Yates T, Biddle SJH et al. Effectiveness of the Stand More AT (SMArT) Work Intervention: cluster randomised controlled trial *BMJ*, 2018; 363:k3870. Doi:10.1136/bmj.k3870

Chapter 16: The Complications of Exercise

1. Royal S. Copeland. Play Safe in Taking Physical Exercise. *Chester Times*, 26 June1926

2. Maron BJ, Doerer JJ, Haas TS et al. Sudden deaths in young competitive athletes: analysis of 1866 deaths in the United States, 1980–2006. *Circulation*, 2009; 119:1085–92

3. Malhotra A, Dhutia H, Finocchario G et al. Outcome of screening in adolescent soccer players. *N Engl J Med*, 2018; 379:524–34

4. Semsarian C, Sweeting J, Ackerman M. Sudden cardiac death in athletes. *Brit Med J*, 2015; 350:h1218

5. Landry CH, Allan KS, Connelly KA et al. Sudden cardiac arrest during participation in competitive sports. *N Eng J Med*, 2017; 377:1943–53

6. Harris KM, Creswell LL, Haas TS et al. Death and Cardiac Arrest in U.S. Triathlon Participants, 1985 to 2016: A Case Series. *Ann Intern Med*, 2017; 167(8):529–35

7. James J, Merghani A, Sharma S. Sudden death in Marathon runners. *Cardiac Electrophysiol Clin*, 2013; 5:43–51

8. Kamil-Rosenberg S, Kokkinos P, de Sousa e Silva C et al. Association between cardiorespiratory fitness, obesity, and incidence of atrial fibrillation. *IJC Heart & Vasculature*, 2020; 31, 100663

9. Abdulla J, Nielsen JR. Is the risk of atrial fibrillation higher in athletes than in the general population? A systematic review and meta-analysis. *Europace*, 2009; 11:1156–9

10. Elliott A, Linz D, Mishima R et al. Association between physical activity and risk of incident arrhythmias in 402 406 individuals: evidence from the UK Biobank cohort. *European Heart Journal*, 2020; 41: 1479–86. https://doi.org/10.1093/eurheartj/ehz897

11. George K, Spence A, Naylor L et al. Cardiac adaptation to acute and chronic participation in endurance sports. *Heart*, 2011; 97:1999–2004

12. DeFina L, Radford N, Barlow C et al. Association of all-cause and cardiovascular mortality with high levels of physical activity and concurrent coronary artery calcification. *JAMA Cardiol*, 2019; 4(2):174–81. Doi: 10.1001/jamacardio.2018.4628

13. Haskell W, I-Min Lee, Pate R et al. Physical activity and public health. Updated recommendations for adults from the American College for Sports Medicine and the American Heart Association. *Circulation*, 2007; 116:1081–93

14. Heesch KC, Miller YD, Brown WJ. Relationship between physical activity and stiff or painful joints in mid-aged women and older women: a 3-year prospective study. *Arthritis Res Ther*, 2007; 9(2):R34

15. Ageberg E, Engstrom G, Gerhardsson de Verdier M et al. Effect of leisure time physical activity on severe knee or hip osteoarthritis

leading to total joint replacement: a population-based prospective cohort study. *BMC Musculoskelet Disord*, 2012; 13:73

16. Hootman JM, Macera CA, Helmick CG, Blair SN. Influence of physical activity-related joint stress on the risk of self-reported hip/knee osteoarthritis: a new method to quantify physical activity. *Prev Med*, 2003; 36:636–44

17. Dunsky A, Netz Y. Physical Activity and Sport in Advanced Age: Is it Risky? – A Summary of Data from Articles Published Between 2000-2009. *Current Aging Science*, 2012; 5:66–71

18. Uusi-Rasi K, Patil R, Karinkanta S et al. Exercise and Vitamin D in Fall Prevention Among Older Women: A Randomized Clinical Trial. *JAMA Intern Med*, 2015; 175:703–11

19. Welsh C, Celis-Morales C, Ho F et al. Association of injury related hospital admissions with commuting by bicycle in the UK: prospective population based study. *BMJ*, 2020; 368:m336 http://dx.doi.org/10.1136/bmj.m336

20. Stewart W. Sport associated dementia. *BMJ*, 21 January 2021; 372:n168. Doi: 10.1136/bmj.n168. PMID: 33478970

21. Abbasi J. Concussions Linked With Erectile Dysfunction in Football Player Study. *JAMA*, 18 February 2020; 323(7):597–8. Doi: 10.1001/jama.2019.21883. PMID: 31995138

22. Lavie C, Hecht H, Wisloff U. Extreme Physical Activity May Increase Coronary Calcification, But Fitness Still Prevails. *Mayo Clin Proc*, 2019; 3:103–9. https://doi.org/10.1016/j.mayocpiqo.2019.03.007

23. Bumann A, Banzer W, Fleckenstein J. Prevalence of Biopsychosocial Factors of Pain in 865 Sports Students of the Dach (Germany, Austria, Switzerland) Region – A Cross-Sectional Survey. *J Sports Sci Med*, June 2020; 19(2): 323–36

24. Hausenblas HA, Schreiber K, Smoliga JM. Addiction to exercise. *BMJ*, 2017; 375:j1745

25. Slay HA, Hayaki J, Napolitano MA, Brownell KD. Motivations for running and eating attitudes in obligatory versus nonobligatory runners. *Int J Eat Disord*,1998; 357:267–75

Conclusions

1. Brown D, Brown D, Heath G et al. Associations between physical activity dose and health related quality of life. *Med Sci Sports Exerc*, 2004; 36:890–96

2. Chief Medical Officer. *On the state of the public health*. Annual Report of Chief Medical Officer, 2009. www.dh.gov.uk/en/Publicationsandstatistics/Publications/AnnualReports/DH_113912

3. Byberg L, Melhus H, Gedeborg R et al. Total mortality after changes in leisure time physical activity in 50 year old men: 35 year follow-up of population based cohort. *Brit Med J*, 2009; 338:936

4. Miller G, Rejeski W, Reboussin B et al. Physical activity, functional limitations and disability in older adults. *J Am Geriatr Soc*, 2000; 48:1264–72

Acknowledgements

My first thank you is to the wonderful cartoonist Toni Goffe, who has illustrated this book so skilfully and entertainingly. He has lightened the tone of what is sometimes quite a serious read. He has also illustrated my weekly blog over the past two years. I am very grateful, too, to all those who have commented on the blog and so contributed to the book, on which the blog has been based.

Thank you, too, to those who helped me get the book into some sort of order by reading the first drafts and advising me on how they could be improved: Dr Karen O'Reilly, Dr Christopher Everett and Mrs Mary Hopfield.

Very grateful thanks also to the team of librarians at Basingstoke Hospital's Healthcare Library for sending me a regular list of up-to-date references to exercise and always being willing to dig out papers to which I did not otherwise have access.

Brenda Updegraff has edited the manuscript with great skill and attention to detail and made many very helpful suggestions for improvements to the text. Her husband, Robert, has expertly created the design and layout of the book. Just to complete the family's contributions, their daughter Eleanor has read the proofs and sought out the howlers which the rest of us missed, as has my old schoolfriend William Winter. Thank you also to Vicki Robinson for her splendid index.

Finally, very many thanks to my long-suffering wife, Lesley, who has tolerated my long absences when I have been hunched up in the study rather than being a more sociable partner. To her I dedicate this book – she is never on the couch very long.

Hugh Bethell, October 2021

Index

CPSIA information can be obtained
at www.ICGtesting.com
Printed in the USA
BVHW060305291221
625052BV00029B/2159